PROFESSIONAL SERVICES FOR MEN:
FACIAL MASSAGE, SHAVING, AND HAIR DESIGN

THOMSON

DELMAR LEARNING

Australia   Canada   Mexico   Singapore   Spain   United Kingdom   United States

THOMSON
★
DELMAR LEARNING

Milady's Professional Services for Men: Facial Massage, Shaving, and Hair Design

President, Milady:
Dawn Gerrain

Director of Learning Solutions:
Sherry Dickinson

Acquisitions Editor:
Brad Hanson

Product Manager:
Erik Herman

Editorial Assistant:
Jessica Burns

Director of Content and Media Productions:
Wendy A. Troeger

Content Project Manager:
Nina Tucciarelli

Associate Content Project Manager:
Angela Iula

Composition:
Carlisle Publishing Services

Director of Marketing:
Wendy Mapstone

Marketing Channel Manager:
Sandra Bruce

Marketing Coordinator:
Nicole Riggi

Cover Design:
Essence of Seven

Library of Congress Cataloging-in-Publication Data:
Milady's professional services for men : facial massage, shaving, and hair design.
  p. cm. — (Professional services for men)
Includes index.
ISBN-10: 1-4180-5084-9
ISBN-13: 978-1-4018-8169-6
1. Barbering. I. Milady Publishing Company. II. Title: Facial massage, shaving, and hair design. III. Series.
TT957.M55154 2007
646.7'24—dc22

2006016059

NOTICE TO THE READER

Publisher does not warrant or guarantee any of the products described herein or perform any independent analysis in connection with any of the product information contained herein. Publisher does not assume, and expressly disclaims, any obligation to obtain and include information other than that provided to it by the manufacturer.

The reader is expressly warned to consider and adopt all safety precautions that might be indicated by the activities herein and to avoid all potential hazards. By following the instructions contained herein, the reader willingly assumes all risks in connection with such instructions.

The publisher makes no representation or warranties of any kind, including but not limited to the warranties of fitness for particular purpose or merchantabiity, nor are any such representations implied with respect to the material set forth herein, and the publisher takes no responsibility with respect to such material. The publisher shall not be liable for any special, consequential, or exemplary damages resulting, in whole or part, from the readers' use of, or reliance upon, this material.

TABLE OF CONTENTS

SHAVING AND FACIAL HAIR DESIGN / 55

2

PREFACE

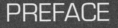

resurgence of barbers, barbershops, and barbering is taking place nationwide as the male consumer once again seeks the ambience and services of a real barbershop. To meet the growing needs and demands of their male clientele, many shops are finding they must offer a full range of professional hair and skin care services for men—it is no longer enough to offer just a good cut. Have you found yourself in this position? Are you an experienced barber who needs to learn more about male skin care and facial hair design? Are you interested in managing your own shop? Do you know all there is to know about cutting and styling but find hair coloring or hair restoration are new to you? Do you want to add men's services to your salon or day spa and need information specific to caring for male clientele? Or, are you new to the profession and want to learn about the fundamentals of cutting and styling, or seek a barbering position? Whatever the case may be, the *Professional Services for Men* series is for you.

Thomson Delmar Learning has created a series of concise, informative books designed to help licensed barbers and stylists develop the skills necessary to meet the growing needs of their male clientele. The four books in the series are:

Professional Services for Men: Facial Massage, Shaving, and Hair Design

Professional Services for Men: Haircoloring and Hair Restoration

Professional Services for Men: Haircutting and Styling

Professional Services for Men: Career Management for Barbers

Each book presents the need-to-know information in an easy to understand format. Utilizing numerous full-color images and drawings, straightforward language, and helpful features such as "Tech Terms," "FYI," "Caution," and "Focus On," for added learning enrichment in your profession. To enhance your learning, the first three books take you step-by-step through the fundamental techniques of hair and skin care for men while emphasizing client comfort and safety. The last book in the *Professional Services for Men* series moves away from the technical aspects of providing men's services and looks toward the career management side of the profession.

It is estimated that 15 to 20 percent of the skin care clientele in spas and salons is male, and that percentage is expected to grow in the future. These men are seeking the physiologically and psychologically rewarding experience of hot steam towels, shaves, and facials provided in a comfortable and relaxing environment. *Professional Services for Men: Facial Massage and Hair Design* is designed to help you develop or sharpen the skills necessary to provide such services. In *Section 1, Men's Facial Massage and Treatments,* you will find the basics about *facial massage, facial treatments,* and the *various types of facials.* You will also find information on *skins types, skin analysis,* and the *equipment* used to provide massage treatments. In *Section 2, Shaving and Facial Hair Design,* you will discover the fundamentals of shaving, including information on the *14 different shaving areas,* the *four standard shaving positions and strokes, how to prepare the client for shaving,* and *how to perform the neck shave.* You will also learn the basics of *how to trim and design a mustache and beard.*

So, if you want to learn about facial massage, shaving, and facial hair design, or want to brush up on your skills in these areas, don't delay—turn the page and let's begin!

A very special thank you to the following individuals for their contributions and assistance with the Professional Men's Services series:

Maura T. Scali-Sheahan, Master Barber and Educator
Cory Cole, Master Barber
Vinny Federico, Master Barber
Laura Downs, Barber
Greg Zorian, Jr., Master Barber
Greg Zorian, III, Master Barber
Helen Wos, Instructor/Barber
Lorilee Bird, Student Barber
Mark Blue, Student Barber
Christopher Morris, Student Barber
Kristen Santa Lucia, Student Barber

Andis, William Marvy Company, Wahl, and 44/20 for use of their product photographs.

Gregory's Barbershop, Clifton Park, NY for use of their location.

Photography Credits:

Section 1: Section Opener, Figures 1–7, 32–38, Paul Castle Photography
Section 2: Section Opener, Figures 39–106, Paul Castle Photography

PROFESSIONAL SERVICES FOR MEN:
FACIAL MASSAGE, SHAVING, AND HAIR DESIGN

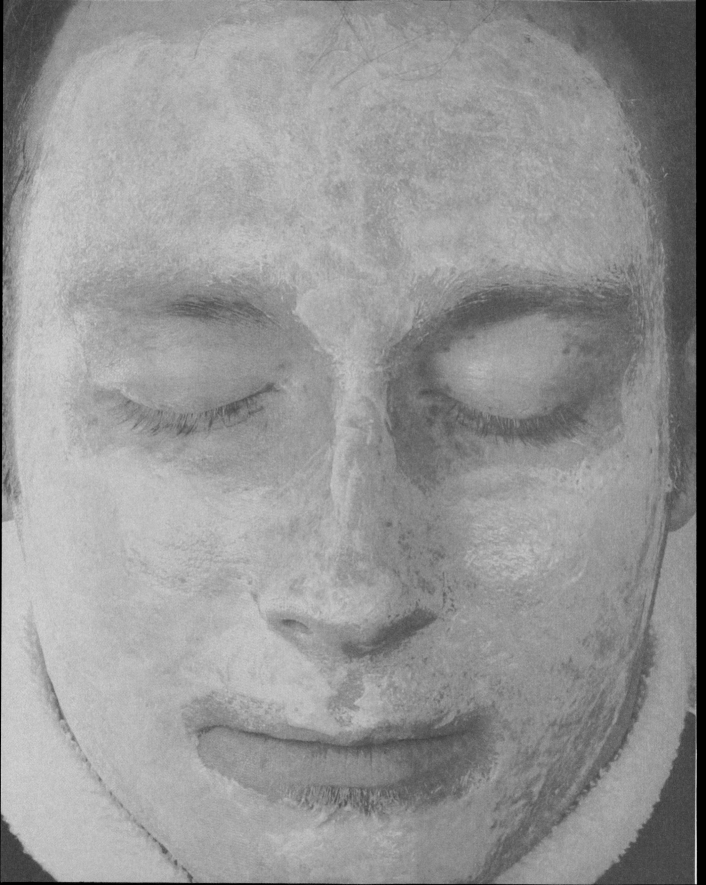

MEN'S FACIAL MASSAGE
AND TREATMENTS

1

A facial massage and treatment is one of the most relaxing and restful services offered in the barbershop. When performed correctly, regularly scheduled facials can produce noticeable improvement in the client's skin tone, texture, and appearance. To perform a professional facial, barbers must be able to analyze skin conditions and recommend the most effective treatments. The development of these abilities begins with a basic knowledge of the anatomical structure of the head, face, and neck; primary subdermal systems; and the theory of massage.

■ TECH TERM

Subdermal refers to those structures, such as muscles, veins, capillaries, arteries, glands, and so on, that are found below the skin's surface.

■ SUBDERMAL SYSTEMS AND FACIAL MASSAGE

Muscles, nerves, and arteries of the head, face, and neck are three of the subdermal systems associated with the performance of facial treatments. *Muscles* are fibrous tissues that have the ability to stretch, contract, and produce all body movements. *Nerves* are long, white fibrous cords that act as message carriers from the brain and spinal column to and from all parts of the body. *Arteries* are elastic, muscular, and thick-walled blood vessels that transport blood under very high pressure.

The muscles, nerves, and arteries of the head, face, and neck will all be affected by facial massage and treatments; therefore, it is the barber's responsibility to perform facial services that will prove beneficial to the client.

Stimulation of Muscles

Muscular tissue may be stimulated by any of the following actions:

- Massage (hand massage and electric vibrator)
- Electric current (high-frequency and faradic current)
- Light rays (infrared rays and ultraviolet rays)
- Heat rays (heating lamps and heating caps)
- Moist heat (steamers and moderately warm steam towels)
- Nerve impulses (through the nervous system)
- Chemicals (certain acids and salts)

Muscles Affected by Massage

The barber or stylist is concerned with the voluntary muscles of the head, face, and neck. It is essential to know the location of these muscles, as well as what they control. Table 1 provides a summary of the muscles of the head, face, and neck.

Stimulation of Nerves

Stimulation to the nerves causes muscles to expand and contract. Heat and moist heat on the skin cause relaxation and cold causes contraction.

Nerve stimulation may be accomplished by any of the following means:

- Chemicals (certain acids and salts)
- Massage (hand massage and electric vibrator)
- Electrical current (high-frequency)
- Light rays (infrared)
- Heat rays (heating lamps and heating caps)
- Moist heat (steamers and moderately warm steam towels)

■ TECH TERM

Faradic current is alternating current that produces a mechanical reaction without chemical effects.

Table 1		MUSCLES OF THE HEAD, FACE, AND NECK

MUSCLE	LOCATION	FUNCTION
Epicranius (occipito-frontalis)	Scalp	a broad muscle that covers the top of the skull
Frontalis	Scalp	the front portion of the epicranius that draws the scalp forward and causes wrinkles across the forehead
Occipitalis	Scalp	muscle at the back part of the epicranius that draws the scalp backward
Aponeurosis	Scalp	tendon that connects the occipitalis and the frontalis
Orbicularis oculi	Eyebrows	completely surrounds the margin of the eye socket; closes the eyelid
Corrugator	Eyebrows	muscle beneath the frontalis and orbicularis oculi that draws the eyebrows down and in; produces vertical lines and causes frowning
Procerus	Nose	covers the top of the nose, depresses the eyebrow, and causes wrinkles across the bridge of the nose; the other nasal muscles are small muscles around the nasal openings, which contract and expand the opening of the nostrils
Levator labii superioris (quadratus labii superioris)	Mouth	a muscle surrounding the upper lip that elevates the upper lip and dilates the nostrils
Depressor labii inferioris (quadratus labii inferioris)	Mouth	a muscle that surrounds the lower part of the lip, depressing the lower lip and drawing it a little to one side
Buccinator	Mouth	muscle between the upper and lower jaws; it compresses the cheeks and expels air between the lips
Levator anguli oris (caninus)	Mouth	raises the angle of the mouth and draws it inward
Mentalis	Mouth	situated at the tip of the chin; it raises and pushes up the lower lip, causing wrinkling of the chin
Orbicularis oris	Mouth	forms a flat band around the upper and lower lips; it compresses, contracts, puckers, and wrinkles the lips

Table 1	CONTINUED	
MUSCLE	**LOCATION**	**FUNCTION**
Risorius	Mouth	extends from the masseter muscle to the angle of the mouth; it draws the corner of the mouth out and back
Zygomaticus	Mouth	extends from the zygomatic bone to the angle of the mouth; elevates the lip
Triangularis	Mouth	extends along the side of the chin; draws down the corner of the mouth
Auricularis superior	Ears	muscle above the ear that draws it upward
Auricularis posterior	Ears	muscle behind the ear that draws it backward
Auricularis anterior	Ears	muscle in front of the ear that draws it forward
Masseter and the temporalis	Mastrication muscles	muscle that coordinate in opening and closing the mouth; are sometimes referred to as chewing muscles
Platysma	Neck, chest, and shoulders	broad muscle extending from the chest and shoulder muscles to the side of the chin; responsible for depressing the lower jaw and lip
Sternocleidomastoideus	Neck, chest, to back of ear	extends from the collar and chest bones to the temporal bone in back of the ear; bends and rotates the head
Trapezius	Neck and shoulders	allows movement of the shoulders and covers the back of the neck

Nerves Affected by Facial Massage

There are 12 pairs of cranial nerves and all are connected to a part of the brain surface. The cranial nerves of most interest in the performance of facial and scalp treatments are the fifth, seventh, and eleventh cranial nerves. Cranial nerves are numbered according to the order in which they emerge from the brain and are named by the description of their nature or function. Table 2 provides a review of the nerves of the head, face, and neck.

| Table 2 | CRANIAL NERVES AFFECTED BY FACIAL MASSAGE |

CRANIAL NERVE	NAME	TYPE	CONTROLS
First	Olfactory	Sensory	sense of smell
Second	Optic	Sensory	sense of sight
Third	Oculomotor	Motor	motion of the eye
Fourth	Trochlear	Motor	upward/downward motion of the eye
Fifth	Trigeminal or Trifacial	Sensory-Motor	sensations of the face, tongue, and teeth
Chief sensory nerve of the face and motor nerve to muscles of mastication	Supraorbital: affects the skin of the forehead, scalp, eyebrows, and upper eyelids Supratrochlear: affects the skin between the eyes and upper sides of the nose Infratrochlear: affects the membrane and skin of the nose Nasal: affects the point and lower sides of the nose Zygomatic: affects the skin of the temples, sides of the forehead, and upper part of the cheeks Infraorbital: affects the skin of the lower eyelids, and sides of the nose, upper lip, and mouth Auriculotemporal: affects the external ear and the skin from above the temples to the top of the skull Mental: affects the skin of the lower lip and chin		
Sixth	Abducent	Motor	motion of the eye
Seventh	Facial	Sensory-motor	motion of the face, scalp, neck, ear, and sections of the palate and tongue
Chief motor nerve of the face	Posterior auricular: affects muscles behind the ears at the base of the skull Temporal: affects the muscles of the temples, sides of the forehead, eyebrows, eyelids, and upper part of the cheeks Zygomatic affects the muscles of the upper part of the cheeks Buccal: affects the muscles of the mouth Mandibular: affects the muscles of the chin and lower lip Cervical: affects the sides of the neck		

Table 2	CONTINUED

CRANIAL NERVE	NAME	TYPE	CONTROLS
Eighth	Acoustic	Sensory	sense of hearing
Ninth	Glossopharyngeal	Sensory-motor	sense of taste
Tenth	Vagus	Sensory-motor	motion and sensations of the ear, pharynx, larynx, heart, lungs, and esophagus
Eleventh	Accessory	Motor	motion of the neck muscles
	Spinal branch: affects the muscles of the neck and back		
Twelfth	Hypoglossal	Motor	motion of the tongue

Spinal or cervical nerves can also be affected by facial massage. The cervical nerves originate at the spinal cord and their branches supply the muscles and scalp at the back of the head and neck, as shown in Table 3.

Table 3	CRANIAL NERVES AFFECTED BY FACIAL MASSAGE

NERVE	LOCATION	FUNCTION
Greater occipital	back of the head	affects the scalp as far up as the top of the head
Lesser occipital	base of the skull	affects the scalp and muscles of this region
Greater auricular	side of the neck	affects the external ears and the areas in front and back of the ears
Cutaneous colli	side of the neck	affects the front and sides of the neck, as far down as the breastbone

Arteries Affected by Facial Massage

An artery is a tubular, thick-walled, elastic vessel that, like capillaries and veins, is part of the circulatory system that transports blood from the heart to all parts of the body. Blood returns to the heart through the veins. The primary arteries that are affected by facial massage are presented in Table 4.

Veins Affected by Facial Massage

The deoxygenated blood returning to the heart from the head, face, and neck flows on each side of the neck in two principal veins: the internal jugular and the external jugular. The most important veins are parallel to the arteries and take the same names as the arteries. Both the internal and external jugular veins serve the areas of head, face, neck, and chest.

THEORY OF MASSAGE

Most clients enjoy a properly administered facial treatment for its stimulating and relaxing effects. Facial massage involves the external manipulation of the face and requires a skillful touch. This is accomplished with the hands, or with the aid of electrical appliances such as electric massagers or vibrators. Each massage movement is executed in such a way as to obtain a specific result.

The benefits of massage depend upon the type, intensity, and extent of the manipulations used. Massage must be performed systematically and never in a casual or irregular manner. The condition of the skin and the general physical condition of the client should always be considered. Normal skin may receive soothing, mildly stimulating, or strongly stimulating massage treatments. Sensitive, inflamed skin could be further damaged, however, by massage. If massage is desired, the manipulations must be gentle and soothing to damaged or sensitive skin. Massage should be used with judgment and moderation.

Table 4	ARTERIES AFFECTED BY FACIAL MASSAGE

ARTERY	ARTERIAL BRANCHES AND BLOOD SUPPLY AREA	
Common carotids Main sources of blood supply to the head, face, and neck; located at the sides of the neck	Internal division: supplies the brain, eye sockets, eyelids, and forehead External division: supplies superficial parts of the head, face, and neck	
External maxillary (facial artery) supplies the lower region of the face, mouth, and nose	Submental: supplies chin and lower lip Inferior labial: supplies lower lip Angular: supplies side of the nose Superior labial: supplies upper lip, septum, and the wings of the nose	
Superficial temporal	Continuation of External Carotid	Supplies muscles, skin, and scalp on the front side, and top of the head
	Frontal	Supplies the forehead
	Parietal	Supplies the crown and sides of the head
	Transverse facial	Supplies the masseter
	Middle temporal	Supplies the temples and eyelids
	Anterior auricular	Supplies the anterior part of the ear
Occipital	Supplies the scalp and back of the head up to the crown	
	Sternocleidomastoideus	Supplies the sternocleidomstoideus muscle
Posterior auricular	Supplies the scalp, behind and above the ear	
	Auricular	Supplies the skin in back of the ear

Massage should never be recommended or employed when the following conditions are present:

- inflammation of the skin
- severe skin lesions
- pus-containing pimples
- high blood pressure
- skin infection

Massage Manipulations

When massaging any part of the head, face, or neck, any pressure should be applied in an upward direction. This rule should be followed in all massage manipulations, whether they are intended to stimulate, relax, or soothe the skin. When applying rotary manipulations, the same rule applies because the pressure should be applied on the upward swing of the movement.

An understanding of the motor points of the face is important in the performance of an effective facial massage. A *motor point* is a point on the skin over a muscle where pressure or stimulation will cause contraction of that muscle. A review of the motor points as illustrated in Figure 1 will assist in the manipulation of the facial muscles during a treatment.

Effleurage is the stroking movement. This is a light, continuous movement applied in a slow and rhythmic manner over the skin with no pressure. The palms are used over large surfaces and the fingertips work the small surfaces, such as around the eyes. Effleurage is frequently used on the forehead, face, and scalp for its soothing and relaxing effects.

To correctly position the fingers for the stroking movement, slightly curve the fingers with just the cushions of the fingertips touching the skin (Figure 2). Do not use the ends of the fingertips for these massage movements. Because the tips of the fingers are pointier than the cushions, the fingernails may scratch the client's skin.

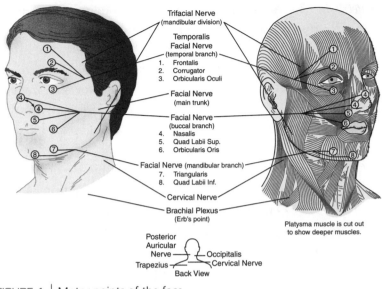

FIGURE 1 | Motor points of the face.

To correctly position the palms for the stroking movement, hold your hands loosely and keep your wrist and fingers flexible. Curve your fingers and palms to conform to the shape of the area being massaged (Figure 3).

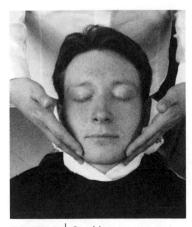

FIGURE 2 | Stroking movement with the fingertips.

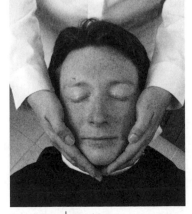

FIGURE 3 | Stroking movements with the palms.

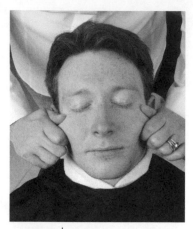

FIGURE 4 | Pétrissage.

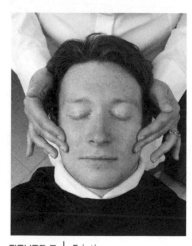

FIGURE 5 | Friction.

Pétrissage is the kneading movement performed with a light, firm pressure. In this movement, the skin and flesh are grasped between the thumb and fingers. As the tissues are lifted from their underlying structures they are squeezed, rolled, or pinched with a light, firm pressure. Pétrissage exerts an invigorating effect on the part being treated and kneading movements give deeper stimulation to the muscles, nerves, and skin glands, and improve the circulation.

Although kneading movements are usually used on large surfaces such as the shoulders and back, digital kneading can be used on the cheeks with light pinching movements (Figure 4).

Friction is a deep rubbing movement in which pressure is applied on the skin while moving it over an underlying structure. The fingers or palms are employed to perform light circular friction on the face and neck. Friction has proven beneficial to the circulation and glandular activity of the skin (Figure 5).

Percussion or *tapotement* consists of short and quick tapping, slapping, or hacking movements. This form of massage is the most stimulating and should be used with care and discretion. Tapping movements are gentler than slapping movements. Percussion movements tone the muscles and impart a healthy glow to the part being massaged.

In tapping, the fingertips are brought down against the skin in rapid succession with even force (Figure 6). In slapping movements, the palm is used to lightly strike the skin. One hand follows the other and slightly lifts the skin with each slapping stroke. Hacking movements employ the outer edges of the hands, which are struck against the skin in alternate succession, and are usually used on the back and shoulders.

Vibration is a rapid shaking movement that can be performed with the fingertips or an electric massager or vibrator. Both methods are used to transmit a trembling movement to the skin and its underlying structures. To prevent overstimulation, this movement should be used sparingly and should never exceed a few seconds' duration on any one spot (Figure 7).

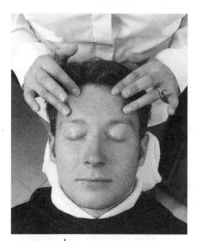

FIGURE 6 | Percussion.

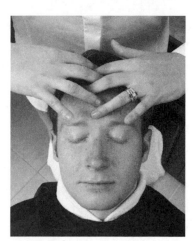

FIGURE 7 | Vibration.

Physiological Effects of Massage

Skillfully applied massage influences the structures and functions of the body, either directly or indirectly. The immediate effect of massage is first noticed on the skin. The part being massaged reacts with an increase in its functional activities, such as more active circulation, secretion, nutrition, and excretion. There is scarcely an organ of the body that is not affected favorably by scientific massage treatments. Beneficial results that may be obtained by proper massage include:

- The skin and all its structures are nourished.
- Muscle fiber is stimulated and strengthened.
- Fat cells are reduced.
- Circulation of blood is increased.
- The activity of the skin and scalp glands is stimulated.
- The skin is rendered soft and pliable.
- The nerves are soothed and rested.
- Pain is sometimes relieved.

Facial Massage Manipulations

When performing facial massage manipulations, remember that an even tempo or rhythm induces relaxation. Once the manipulations have begun, one or both of the hands should remain on the skin at all times. When it becomes necessary to remove the hands, avoid abrupt motions and gently feather-off the hands from the skin.

Remember that massage movements are directed from the insertion toward the origin of a muscle to avoid damage to muscular tissues. Refer to Figure 1 and apply minimal pressure on the motor points of the face when performing the massage manipulations described in the next sections.

▷ procedure no. 1

Massage Manipulation

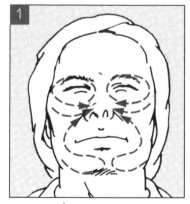

FIGURE 8 | Applying cleansing cream.

Figures 8 through 16 show the direction of different massage movements that may be used on the various parts of the face and neck. You may employ a massage manipulation procedure that is equally correct.

1 Apply cleansing cream lightly over the face with stroking, spreading, and circulatory movements (Figure 8).

2 Stroke fingers across forehead with up-and-down movements (Figure 9).

3 Manipulate fingers across the forehead with a circular movement (Figure 10).

4 Stroke fingers upward along sides of nose (Figure 11).

5 Apply a circular movement over sides of nose and use a light, stroking movement around the eyes (Figure 12).

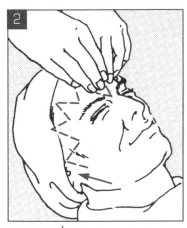

FIGURE 9 | Using up-and-down movements across forehead.

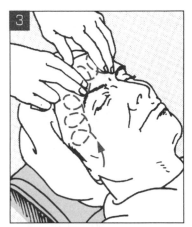

FIGURE 10 | Circular movement across the forehead.

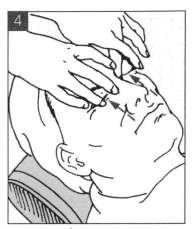

FIGURE 11 | Stroking movement along side of nose.

6 Manipulate the temples, and then the front and back of the ears, with a wide circular movement (Figure 13).

7 Gently stroke both thumbs across upper lip (Figure 14).

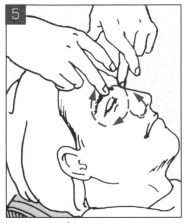

FIGURE 12 | A combination of circular and stroking movements.

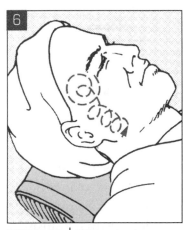

FIGURE 13 | Wide, circular movements in the temple area.

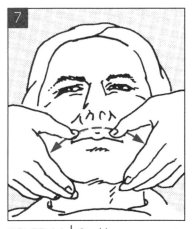

FIGURE 14 | Stroking movement across the upper lip.

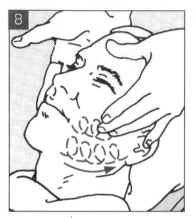

FIGURE 15 | Rotary circular movements on the lower face.

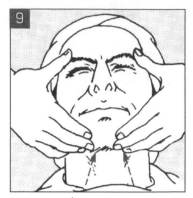

FIGURE 16 | Manipulating fingers from under chin to back of ears to temples.

i **FYI**

Massage manipulations on the face are usually performed with upward movements; however, the presence of facial hair may require a different approach. Gently direct massage movements in the direction of beard growth. Massage manipulations that go against or across the grain may cause discomfort to the client.

■ TECH TERM

Electrical modalities are currents used in electric facial and scalp treatments.

8   Manipulate fingers from the corners of the mouth to the cheeks and temples with a rotary (circular) movement. Manipulate fingers along the lower jaw from the tip of the chin to the ear using the same technique (Figure 15).

9   Stroke fingers above and below lower jawbone from the chin to the ear. Manipulate fingers from under the chin and neck to the back of the ears and up to the temples (Figure 16).

■ EQUIPMENT FOR MASSAGE TREATMENTS

In addition to massage techniques performed with the hands, appliances such as massagers or vibrators, brush machines, electrical modalities, and light rays can be used to enhance the facial treatment service.

The *electric massager* most often used in barbershops is a handheld unit that transmits vibrations through the barber's hand to the client's skin and muscles (Figure 17). This type of massaging technique is used over heavy muscle tissue such as

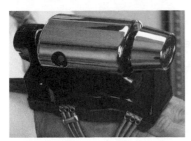

FIGURE 17 │ Handheld massager.

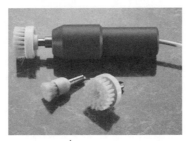

FIGURE 18 │ The brush machine helps cleanse and lightly exfoliate the skin.

the scalp and shoulders to produce a succession of stimulating impulses. It has an invigorating effect on muscle tissue, increases the blood supply to the parts treated, is soothing to the nerves, increases glandular activity, and stimulates the skin and scalp. When used correctly, electric massagers can be used to perform vibratory facials.

The *brush machine* helps to stimulate, cleanse, and lightly exfoliate the skin. Many different models are available from a variety of manufacturers. Typically these units have two or three small brush attachments that can be rotated at different speeds (Figure 18).

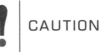 **CAUTION**

Some hand-massager appliances are heavy and cumbersome for smaller hands. Always "try one on for size" before purchasing.

 procedure no. 2

Using a Rotary Brush Machine

The procedure for using a rotary brush machine is as follows:

1 Perform a light cleansing on the skin.

2 Insert the appropriate size brush for the face into the handheld device.

3 Apply more cleanser to the skin.

4 Dip the brush into water and begin the pattern of movement at the forehead.

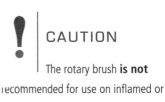 **CAUTION**

The rotary brush **is not** recommended for use on inflamed or acne-prone skin.

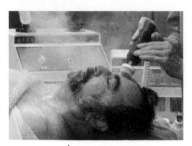

FIGURE 19 | To properly use the brush machine, a light touch is used, with no pressure on the skin.

■ TECH TERM

Antiseptic means any substance that inhibits the action of microorganisms.

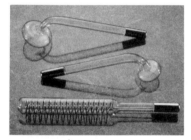

FIGURE 20 | Electrodes for the high-frequency machine.

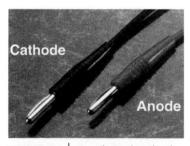

FIGURE 21 | Anode and cathode.

5   Continue the rotation down the cheeks, nose, upper lip, chin, jaw, and neck areas. No pressure should be applied, with the bristles of the brush remaining straight (Figure 19).

6   Remoisten the brush as needed during the process. Dryer skin types require a slow, steady rotation. Thicker, oily skin types can tolerate a faster speed.

Steamers are electrical devices that produce and project moist, uniform steam that can be positioned over sections of the head or face for softening and cleansing purposes. The steam warms the skin, inducing the flow of both oil and sweat, and has an antiseptic effect for problematic skin.

Steamers may be used in place of hot towels for scalp and hair reconditioning treatments. When positioned over the scalp, the steam softens the skin, increases perspiration, and promotes the effectiveness of applied scalp tonics and lotions.

Facial treatments performed with *electric facial machines* are a form of electrotherapy. Several electrical currents, or modalities, are used in electrotherapy: high-frequency, galvanic, faradic, and sinusoidal currents. Some electric facial machines can generate all four currents and others may produce only one or two.

Electrical modality machines require an electrode to apply and direct the current to the client's skin. Except for the high-frequency modality (Figure 20), each of the currents requires two electrodes, one positive and one negative, to conduct the flow of electricity through the body. A positive electrode (anode) is red and a negative electrode (cathode) is black, with plus- and minus-sign markings, respectively (Figure 21). Consult the equipment manufacturer for specialized training in the use of the machine.

Light rays are used to impart light-therapy treatments on the skin. Infrared, ultraviolet, white, blue, and red rays are used to produce different effects through the use of therapeutic lamps. Single-function and combination units are available in floor and tabletop models. Table 5 provides a summary of the types of light used in treatments and their beneficial effects.

Table 5	EFFECTS OF LIGHT THERAPY

TYPE OF LIGHT	BENEFICIAL EFFECTS
Ultraviolet	Increases the elimination of waste products Improves the flow of blood and lymph Has a germicidal and antibacterial effect Produces vitamin D in the skin Can be used to treat rickets, psoriasis, and acne Produces a tan
Infrared	Heats and relaxes the skin Dilates blood vessels and increases circulation Produces chemical changes Increases metabolism Increases production of perspiration and oil Deep penetration relieves pain in sore muscles Soothes nerves
White Light	Relieves pain in the back of the neck and shoulders Produces some chemical and germicidial effects Relaxes muscles
Blue Light	Soothes nerves Improves skin tone Provides some chemical and germicidal effects Used for mild cases of skin eruptions Produces little heat
Red Light	Improves dry, scaly, wrinkled skin Relaxes muscles Penetrates the deepest Produces the most heat

High-Frequency Machines

High-frequency or Tesla current is characterized by a high rate of oscillation that is used for both scalp and facial treatments. Although it is sometimes called the *violet ray* because of its color, there are no ultraviolet rays in high-frequency current.

■ TECH TERM

Oscillating current is current that varies regularly between minimum and maximum values.

■ TECH TERM

Thermal means heat.

■ TECH TERM

Metabolism is a complex chemical process whereby cells are nourished and supplied with the energy needed to carry out their activities.

! | CAUTION

When performing electrotherapy treatments, the barber and the client must avoid contact with metals or water.

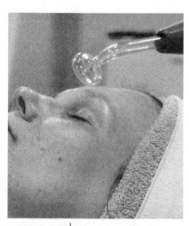

FIGURE 22 | Direct application method using high frequency.

The primary actions of high-frequency current are thermal and antiseptic. Its rapid vibrations do not produce muscular contractions or chemical changes, so the physiological effects are either stimulating or soothing, depending on the method of application.

The electrodes for high-frequency machines are made of glass or metal. Their shapes vary from the flat facial electrode to the rake-shaped scalp electrode. As the current passes through the glass electrode, tiny violet sparks are emitted. All high-frequency treatments should be started with a mild current, which is gradually increased to the required strength. The length of the treatment depends on the condition to be treated. For general facial or scalp treatments, no more than five minutes should be allowed.

The high-frequency machine is a versatile tool that can benefit the client's skin in the following ways:

- stimulates blood circulation
- helps to oxygenate the skin
- increases glandular activity
- aids in elimination and absorption
- increases cell metabolism
- promotes antiseptic and germicidal action
- generates a warm feeling that has a relaxing effect on the skin

Application of High-Frequency Current

For proper use, follow the instructions provided by the manufacturer. Three methods of using Tesla high-frequency current are available: direct surface application, indirect application, and general electrification.

Direct surface application is performed with the mushroom or rake-shaped electrodes for its calming and germicidal effect on the skin (Figure 22). The heat that is generated has a sedative effect, and oily and acne-prone skin benefit from its germicidal action. The germicidal benefits of high-frequency current are produced only with the direct application method. This method can be used on clean, dry skin, over facial creams, and over gauze for a sparking effect.

When applying high-frequency current to the face using the facial electrodes, movements are started on the neck and worked upward to the jaw, cheeks, chin, nose, and forehead.

▷ procedure no. 3

Direct Surface Application of High-Frequency Current

The procedure for direct surface application during a facial treatment is as follows:

1. Place the mushroom-shaped electrode into the handheld device.

2. Adjust the rheostat to the proper setting. If in doubt, start at the lowest setting and increase as needed.

3. Place an index finger on the glass electrode.

4. Apply the electrode directly to the client's skin, beginning on the neck.

5. Glide the electrode over the skin in circular, upward movements on the neck toward the jaw, then cheeks, chin, nose, and forehead areas.

   NOTE: If the electrode tends to drag, place gauze between the skin and the electrode.

6. To remove from the skin, place an index finger over the glass and remove it. Turn the power switch off.

Indirect application is performed with the client holding the wire glass electrode between both hands (Figure 23). To prevent shock, the power is turned on after the client is holding the electrode firmly and is turned off before the electrode is removed from the client's hand. At no time is the electrode held

> **■ TECH TERM**
>
> A *rheostat* is an adjustable resistor used for controlling current in a circuit.

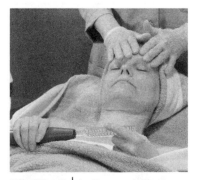

FIGURE 23 | Indirect application method using high frequency.

by the barber or stylist. Indirect application of the current produces both a toning and stimulating effect on the skin that is ideal for aging and sallow skin.

▷ procedure no. 4

Indirect Application of High-Frequency Current

The procedure for indirect application during a facial treatment is as follows:

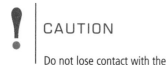

CAUTION

Do not lose contact with the client's skin during this procedure while the current is on.

1 Apply cream to client's face.

2 Instruct the client to hold the wire glass electrode with both hands.

3 The barber places the fingers of one hand on the client's forehead.

4 With the opposite hand, the barber turns the high-frequency machine on to a low setting.

5 Using both hands, the barber performs tapping (tapotement or percussion) motions in a systematic manner over the client's face.

6 To discontinue the high-frequency service, the barber removes one hand from the skin and turns the power off.

reminder

When using high-frequency current, never use a skin or scalp lotion that contains alcohol prior to the electrical treatment, as doing so may cause a fire.

General electrification is performed with the client holding a metal electrode. This method charges the client's body with electricity without being touched by the barber. Calm, sedative, or soothing effects are produced with the general electrification method of application.

SANITIZING AND MAINTENANCE After each use, clean the glass electrode by *wiping* it with a soap and water solution. Do not immerse the electrode directly in water. Next, place only the end of the electrode into a disinfectant solution for 20 minutes.

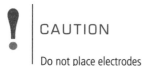

CAUTION

Do not place electrodes in an ultraviolet-ray cabinet sanitizer or autoclave.

Rinse with cool water, but do not get the metal parts wet. Dry with a clean towel and store in a covered container.

Galvanic Machine

The galvanic machine converts the oscillating current received from an outlet into a direct current (Figure 24). The electrons then flow continuously in the same direction. This produces a relaxation response that can be regulated to target specific nerve endings in the epidermis. Galvanic current is used to produce chemical (disincrustation) and ionic (iontophoresis) reactions in the skin. This treatment is beneficial for oily or acne-prone skin.

The galvanic machine has two poles, a negative (−) and a positive (+). Both are used for different effects (Table 6). Several types of electrodes are available for the galvanic machine. The most popular are the disincrustator and the ionizing roller. To make proper contact, each electrode must be covered with cotton and the client must hold the opposite pole electrode.

Applications of Galvanic Current

Disincrustation is used to facilitate deep pore cleansing. During this process, the galvanic current is used to create a chemical reaction that helps to emulsify or liquefy sebum and waste. To perform disincrustation, an acid-based solution is placed onto the skin's surface. When this current passes through certain solutions containing acids and salts, or passes through the tissues and fluids of the body, it produces chemical changes.

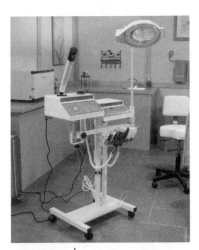

FIGURE 24 | "Five-in-one" machine, including galvanic electrodes.

■ TECH TERM

Direct current is a constant current that travels in one direction only and produces a chemical reaction. *Galvanic current* is a constant and direct current, having a positive and negative pole, that produces chemical changes in tissues and body fluids.

■ TECH TERM

The *epidermis* is the outermost layer of the skin; it is also called the *cuticle* or *scarf skin*.

■ TECH TERM

Sebum is an oily substance secreted by the sebaceous glands. The *sebaceous glands* are the oil glands of the skin, which are connected to hair follicles.

|▷ procedure no. 5

Disincrustation

The procedure for the disincrustation service is as follows:

 Gently cleanse the skin prior to treatment.

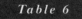

Table 6 | EFFECTS OF POSITIVE AND NEGATIVE POLES

POSITIVE POLE (ANODE)	NEGATIVE POLE (CATHODE)
causes an acid reaction	causes an alkaline reaction
calms or soothes nerve endings	stimulates nerve endings
decreases blood circulation	increases blood circulation; softens and relaxes tissue

2 Instruct the client to remove any jewelry from the hand that will be used to hold the electrode. Cover the electrode held by the client with a moistened sponge or piece of dampened cotton. This electrode is connected to the red wire (positive).

3 Prepare the disincrustator electrode (negative) by placing a dampened sponge or cotton pad into the black ring, then slide the ring back onto the electrode.

4 Dip the electrode into the disincrustation solution and apply the electrode to the client's forehead. Turn the switch to negative and set at 0.05 micro-amps. Gradually turn the rheostat clockwise to increase the intensity of the current. At this point the client will usually experience a metallic taste in the mouth and a slight prickling sensation, which indicate that the current is strong enough. Be sure to explain to the client the sensations he will experience and DO NOT increase the current once these sensations are felt. The alkaline disincrustation solution will be attracted to the positive pole in the client's hand.

5 Gently glide and rotate the electrode over the facial areas that are oily. Before moving the electrode to another section of the face, the current is reduced

back to zero and the process is repeated. The time spent doing the disincrustation part of the facial treatment will depend on the condition of the skin. Anywhere from 3 to 10 minutes may be required for normal to oily and acne-prone skin, respectively.

6 Upon completion, turn the machine off and remove the electrode. Use cotton pads or sponges to rinse the skin with warm water. Proceed with extractions of blackheads and pustules.

Iontophoresis means the introduction of ions. This process uses galvanic current to apply water-soluble solutions into the deeper layers of the skin. The current flows through conductive solutions by means of positive and negative polarities, or ionization. Once the charge of the solution is determined, the machine is set to the appropriate setting. The client holds an electrode with the opposite charge (Figure 25). Moistened sponges or cotton pads are also used in this process.

Phoresis is the process of forcing chemical solutions into unbroken skin by way of a galvanic current. The process of ionic penetration takes place in two forms: cataphoresis and anaphoresis.

Cataphoresis is the use of the positive pole (anode) to introduce an acid pH product, such as an astringent solution, into the skin. Products that have a slightly acid pH are considered positive. The positive pole may also be used to close the follicles or pores after the treatment; decrease redness, as in mild acne; prevent inflammation after blackhead and blemish treatment (decrease blood supply); soothe nerves; and harden tissues.

Anaphoresis is the use of the negative pole (cathode) to force an alkaline pH product, such as disincrustation lotion, into the skin. Products with an alkaline pH are considered to be negative. The negative pole may be used to stimulate the circulation of blood to dry skin, stimulate nerves, and soften tissues. The procedure for ionization is the same as that used in the disincrustation process.

■ TECH TERM

Comedone is another name for a blackhead.

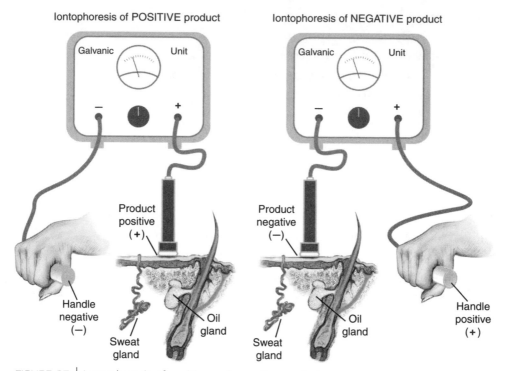

FIGURE 25 | Iontophoresis of positive and negative products.

Ultraviolet-Ray Lamps

Ultraviolet rays are used to treat acne, tinea, seborrhea, and dandruff. Their germicidal effect helps to promote healing and stimulate hair growth. Ultraviolet-ray lamps deliver these shortest light rays of the spectrum. The benefits of these shorter rays are obtained when the lamp is placed 30 to 36 inches from the skin.

Average exposure to ultraviolet rays may produce redness of the skin, and overdoses may cause blistering. It is better to start with a two- or three-minute exposure, and gradually increase the time to seven or eight minutes. The barber must wear tinted safety goggles and the client must wear opaque eye protectors to protect the eyes from the rays.

■ TECH TERM

Tinea is the technical name for ringworm. *Seborrhea* is a skin condition caused by excessive sebum secretion.

Infrared-Ray Lamps

Infrared rays generally produce a soothing and beneficial type of heat that extends for some distance into the tissues of the body. The effects of infrared rays on the exposed skin area include:

- heating and relaxation of the skin without increasing the temperature of the body as a whole

- dilation of blood vessels in the skin and increased blood flow

- increased metabolism and chemical changes within skin tissues

- increased production of perspiration and oil on the skin

- relief of pain

The infrared-ray lamp is operated at an average distance of 30 inches. It is placed closer at the start of the treatment and, in order to avoid burning the skin, is then moved back gradually as the surface heat becomes more pronounced. Always protect the eyes of the client during exposure. Place pads saturated with diluted boric acid or witch hazel solution over the client's eyelids.

Safety Precautions for Using Electrical Equipment

- Disconnect any appliances when they are not being used.

- Study instructions before using any electrical equipment.

- Keep all wires, plugs, and equipment in a safe condition.

- Inspect all electrical equipment frequently.

- Avoid getting electric cords wet.

- Sanitize all electrodes properly.

- Protect the client at all times.

- Do not touch any metal while using electrical appliances.

- Do not handle electrical equipment with wet hands.

- Do not allow the client to touch metal surfaces when electrical treatments are being performed.

- Do not leave the room when the client is attached to any electrical device.

- Do not attempt to clean around an electric outlet when equipment is plugged in.

- Do not touch two metallic objects at the same time while connected to an electric current.

- Do not use any electrical equipment without first obtaining full instruction in its care and use.

The protection and safety of the client are the primary concern of the barber. All electrical equipment should be inspected regularly to determine that it is in good working condition. Carelessness may result in shocks or burns. Barbers who practice safety precautions help to eliminate accidents, assuring greater comfort and satisfaction for their clients.

With a basic knowledge of the anatomical structure of the head, face, and neck and the primary subdermal systems, and the ability to perform massage manipulations manually or with electrical devices, you are now ready to engage in the analysis and performance of skin care.

FACIAL TREATMENTS

The barber does not treat skin diseases but should be able to recognize various skin disorders so as to differentiate between those that can be serviced in the barbershop and those that should be referred to a physician. Facials performed in the barbershop are considered to be either preservative or corrective treatments.

Preservative treatments are intended to help maintain the health of facial skin. The performance of correct cleansing, massage, and electrical treatments can increase circulation, relax the nerves, activate skin glands, and increase cell metabolism.

Corrective treatments are used to correct skin conditions such as dryness, oiliness, blackheads, aging lines, and minor acne. In general, facial treatments are beneficial because they:

- cleanse the skin.
- increase circulation.
- activate glandular activity.
- relax tense nerves.
- maintain muscle tone.
- strengthen weak muscle tissue.
- correct certain skin disorders.
- help prevent the formation of wrinkles and aging lines.
- improve skin texture and complexion.
- help to reduce fatty tissues.

To perform the full range of facial treatments presented in this section, the barber will require access to hot and cold water, soft terry cloth towels, therapeutic lamps, and a variety of preparations designed for facial treatments. These preparations include such items as facial creams, tonics, exfoliants, lotions, oils, packs, and masks.

Skin Types

There are four basic skin types that the barber will need to recognize before the appropriate products can be chosen for a facial treatment. Skin type is primarily based on the amount of oil

■ TECH TERM

Lipids are part of a group of organic compounds consisting of fats and other substances with similar properties. Lipids are not water-soluble, but are soluble in fat solvents and alcohol. Lipids are greasy to the touch and are important cell constituents.

■ TECH TERM

Humectants are substances that help to attract or retain moisture.

that is produced in the follicles from the sebaceous glands and the amount of lipids found between the cells. Skin types include dry, normal, combination, and oily. Any of these skin types can be sensitive to products, irritation, or the environment.

Dry skin does not produce enough oil, which is needed to protect the skin from environmental damage and aging. Dry skin needs extra care because it does not have this protection. The stimulation of oil production and protection of the skin surface is the objective of a facial treatment for dry skin. In some cases, dry skin is also dehydrated skin that lacks water. In addition to drinking plenty of water, hydrating the skin with moisturizers and humectants can help minimize the negative effects of dryness and dehydration.

Normal skin has a good water/oil balance. The follicles are a normal size and the skin is free of blemishes. Maintenance and preservative care is the goal for this type of skin.

Combination skin can be both oily and dry at different areas of the face. The T-zone is the section of the face that incorporates the forehead, nose, and chin area. These areas tend to have more sebaceous glands and larger pores. The cheek and outer areas of the face tend to be dry. Water-based products work best for combination skin types.

Oily skin is characterized by excess sebum production. The follicle size is larger and contains more oil. Oily skin requires more cleansing and exfoliation than other skin types, yet over-cleansing can strip and irritate the skin. If the skin is overdried, it is not balanced and the body will try to produce additional oil to compensate for the dryness on the surface. Proper exfoliation and a water-based hydrator will help keep oily skin clean and balanced.

Wrinkles are depressions in the skin that have developed from repetitious muscle action moving in the same direction. Other factors that influence the formation of wrinkles are:

- loosening of the elastic skin fibers due to abnormal tension or relaxation of the facial muscles

- shrinking of the skin tissue as a result of aging
- excessive dryness of the skin
- improper facial care

Skin Analysis

A knowledge of skin types and conditions is helpful in performing an accurate skin analysis. It is preferable to analyze the skin with a magnifying lamp/light (Figure 26), but if one is not available, a close inspection of the skin will suffice. When analyzing the skin it is important to note the client's skin type and conditions and the skin's visible appearance and texture. Be sure to record this information on a client record card for future use (Figures 27 and 28). Follow guidelines 1–4 when performing a skin analysis:

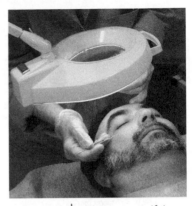

FIGURE 26 | Using a magnifying light to analyze the skin.

CONSULTATION CARD				
Name _____			Date of Consultation _____	
Address _____			D.O.B. _____	
City _____ State _____ Zip _____			Occupation _____	
Tel. (Home) _____ (Business) _____			Ref. by _____	
			Contraindications _____	
Medical History				
Current Medication				
Previous Treatments				
Home Care Products Used				
SKIN TYPE	Oily	Normal	Dry	Combination
SKIN CONDITION	Clogged Pores	Sensitive	Dehydrated	Mature
Skin Abnormalities				
Remarks				

FIGURE 27 | Client consultation card (front).

FACIAL RECORD			
Date	Type of treatment	By	Products purchased
2/14	Cleansing, Peel - Relaxing Massage		Moisturizer with sunscreen
3/16	Cleansing, Peel Modelage Mask		Cleanser, Tonic Lotion
4/5	Cleansing, Peel High Frequency indirect		Moisturizer
4/26	Cleansing, Peel Massage	John	Dry skin cream
5/18	Cleansing, Peel Iontophoresis		
	Skin is showing marked improvement.		
6/1	Cleansing, Peel Relaxing Massage	Mary	

FIGURE 28 │ Client consultation card (back).

1. Observe the client's skin type, condition, and appearance; feel the texture.

2. Ask questions of the client relating to the skin's appearance and home care routine.

3. Discuss the facial procedure and/or treatment plans, the products that will be used, and why.

4. Encourage the client to ask questions and then determine a course of action together.

Skin Care Products

The type of facial treatment will determine the products needed to complete the procedure. Three essential skin care preparations, however, should be used before or after a shave service and during full facial treatments. These essential preparations are cleansers, toners, and moisturizers. Additional products such as exfoliating scrubs, masks, and treatment creams are used in conjunction with the essential preparations during the full facial treatment.

- *Cleansers* should be mild and easy to rinse from the skin. They are available as face washes, lotions, and creams for all types of skin and skin conditions. Face washes are usually water-based products with a neutral or slightly acidic pH effective on oily and combination skin types. Cleansing lotions are water-based emulsions for normal and combination skin that contain emollients or oils to soften the skin. Cleansing creams are oil-based emulsions that are used primarily to dissolve dirt and makeup. Because cleansing creams are heavier than cleansing lotions, performers use these products to remove heavy stage makeup.

- *Toners, fresheners,* and *astringents* are used after cleansing and prior to the application of a moisturizer. These tonic lotions vary in strength and alcohol content and therefore vary in pH.

- Fresheners usually have the lowest alcohol content (0 to 4 percent) and are beneficial for dry, mature, and sensitive skin. Toners are designed to tone or tighten the skin and may be used on normal and combination skin types. The alcohol content range of toners is usually 4 to 15 percent. Astringents may contain up to 35 percent alcohol and are used for oily and acne-prone skin. Toners, fresheners, and astringents all help to remove cleanser residue and have a temporary tightening effect on the skin. Some restore the skin's natural pH after cleansing and others can help certain skin conditions.

- *Moisturizers* are the third essential product needed to perform a facial. Moisturizers are formulated to add moisture to the skin and are available for various skin

i **FYI**

Witch hazel is an astringent commonly used in barbershops.

types. They are also available in water-based and oil-based formulations.

NOTE: The use of cleansers, toners, and moisturizers during the shave service is discussed in Section 2 of this book.

Other types of products are available for specific applications:

- *Exfoliating scrubs* are used to physically rub or remove dead cells from the skin surface. Granular scrubs for normal to dry skin may be used two times per week. Scrubs are available in cream, lotion, and gel forms for a variety of skin types.

- *Masks and packs* draw impurities out of pores, tighten, tone, hydrate, soothe, and nourish the skin, depending on the ingredients. They are available in cream, gel, or clay forms and should be used according to skin type.

Face packs and masks differ in their composition and usage. A mask is usually a setting product, which means that it dries after application, providing complete closure to the environment on top of the skin. Masks are most often applied directly to the skin and are known for their tightening and sebum-absorbing effects. Packs, also referred to as cream or gel masks, are usually applied to the skin over layers of gauze to hold the product in place over the skin. They are beneficial for sensitive skin and have excellent hydrating properties. Applied with a mask brush, they are allowed to set for about 10 minutes.

High-quality packs and masks should feel comfortable while producing slight tingling and tightening sensations. Always follow the manufacturer's directions for preparation, application, and removal of the product from the skin.

Clay masks are clay preparations used to stimulate circulation and temporarily contract the skin pores. They absorb sebum and are used on oily and combination skin types. Applied with a mask brush, they are allowed to set until dry, usually about 10 minutes (Figure 29).

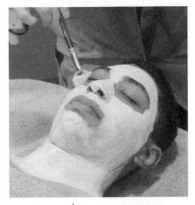

FIGURE 29 | Mask application.

- *Paraffin wax masks* actually employ the pack application method. Specially prepared paraffin is melted at slightly more than body temperature before application. The client's skin is prepared by cleansing, followed by the application of a treatment cream. Eye pads are used and the paraffin is applied over gauze to keep the facial hair from sticking to the wax (Figures 30 and 31).

- Various facial masks and packs are available for use in the barbershop. Hot-oil masks, milk and honey, egg white, and witch hazel packs have been around for many years. For proper use, the barber should always read the manufacturer's claims and directions. When available, attend product information seminars and demonstrations. Judge the merits of the mask or pack before recommending it to a client.

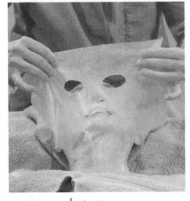

FIGURE 30 | Placing gauze on the client's face.

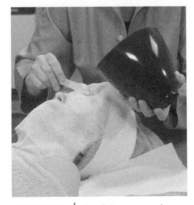

FIGURE 31 | Applying a mask over the gauze.

❑ *Massage creams* are creams, lotions, or oils that provide slip during a massage while also nourishing and treating skin conditions.

❑ *Rolling cream* is a thick, smooth, and usually pink facial cleanser that has been used in barbershops for decades. It is applied in a thin layer over the skin, after which it is rolled off with a firm, stroking motion. As the rolling takes place, loose flaky skin and trapped impurities are lifted from the skin surface. The skin is left soft and smooth with increased circulation to the surface.

In terms of skin care products and the order in which they will be used during full facial treatments in this book, a general outline is as follows:

1. Cleanser

2. Exfoliant (scrub or rolling cream)

3. Massage cream

4. Cleanser

5. Freshener (low alcohol content)

6. Mask

7. Toner or astringent

8. Moisturizer

NOTE: The order in which skin care products are applied may vary from one product line to another, and may also be guided by the policies and procedures of the barbershop.

Men's Skin Care Products

Several decades ago, men's personal care products consisted of basic items such as cologne, hair tonics or creams, deodorants, shaving creams, and aftershave lotions. The high-end versions of these basic items were often created as spin-off products from clothing designers. Even men's hair sprays were almost nonexistent before the 1960s. Today, however, products that have been developed specifically with the male in mind are abundant on retail shelves and in shops and salons. The male consumer is finally getting the attention he deserves and each year more men are experiencing the benefits of using skin care products on a regular basis.

When choosing men's skin care products for use in the barbershop, it is important to think about the specific characteristics of a product that might appeal to men. For example, men in general do not appreciate highly fragranced or multistep products. Creams should be simple, nonfragranced, and absorbent with a matte (non-shiny) finish. Most men do not like the greasy or oily feeling of some products. Men also prefer simpler routines and multipurpose products. For example, a toner that serves as an aftershave will usually be chosen over the purchase and use of two separate products.

Although the quality of the product must be the barber's and the client's first consideration in product choices, packaging characteristics also need to be taken into consideration. Typically, tube packaging is preferred over jars, and size can also be a factor for the client who travels in his profession. One option is to stock barbershop retail shelves with larger containers for the client's home use and smaller, convenient sizes for travel. As a general rule, use the products you retail for services performed within the shop.

NOTE: Smaller packaged goods can also be used for promotions and marketing strategies in the barbershop.

The Basic Facial

The basic facial, sometimes known as the *scientific rest facial,* is beneficial for its cleansing and stimulating action on the skin that also exercises and relaxes the facial muscles. The procedural steps listed next represent one routine that is used to perform a basic facial. It may be changed to conform to your shop's procedures or new procedures that may arise in the industry.

▶ procedure no. 6

Basic Facial

Preparation and performance of a basic facial in the barbershop includes the following steps:

1. Arrange all necessary supplies in a convenient location.

2. Drape the client and engage in client consultation.

3. Perform skin analysis and make product selection.

4. Place a towel or paper barrier between the client's head and the headrest. Adjust the headrest and recline the hydraulic chair. Make sure the client is comfortable.

5. Protect the client's hair with a towel or cap.

6. Wash your hands.

   NOTE: All products should be removed from their containers with a sanitized spatula. Do not dip the fingers into the containers, which may contaminate the product.

7. Apply cleansing cream over the face, using stroking and rotary movements (Figure 32).

8. Remove the cleansing cream with a warm, damp towel (Figure 33).

9. Apply two or three steam towels to open pores and loosen imbedded dirt and oils (Figure 34).

10. Reapply cleansing cream to the skin with the fingertips.

11. Gently massage the face, using continuous and rhythmic movements (Figures 35 and 36).

    NOTE: The brush machine may also be used at this time.

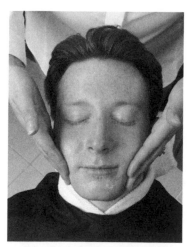

FIGURE 32 | Applying cleansing cream.

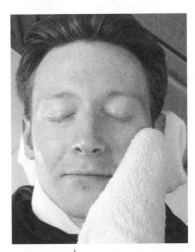

FIGURE 33 | Removing cleansing cream.

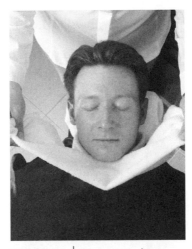

FIGURE 34 | Steam towels.

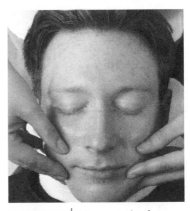

FIGURE 35 | Massage the face.

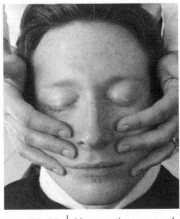

FIGURE 36 | Use continuous and rhythmic movements.

12 Wipe off excess cleansing cream with a warm towel.

13 Apply an exfoliating product and lightly massage over the skin.

14 Apply steam towel. Wipe off excess product until the skin is free of exfoliating residue.

15 Gently wipe toner or astringent over the face, then pat dry (Figure 37).

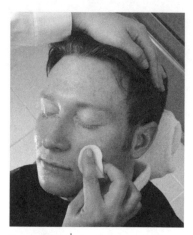

FIGURE 37 | Apply toner or astringent.

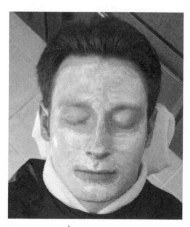

FIGURE 38 | Apply mask; allow to dry.

16 Apply mask or pack and allow to dry (Figure 38).

17 Apply tepid to warm towel to moisten mask/pack. Wipe off product until free of mask/pack.

18 Again, gently wipe toner or astringent over the face and pat dry.

19 Apply a light coat of moisturizer using the effleurage movement.

20 Apply a light dusting of talc if the client desires it. Remove any excess.

21 Slowly raise the hydraulic chair and assist client to a sitting position.

22 Discard all disposable supplies and materials.

23 Wipe containers and close tightly. Store in appropriate place.

24 Sanitize all nondisposable implements and tools.

25 Wash and sanitize your hands.

Points to Remember

- Strive to have the client relax.
- Provide a quiet atmosphere.
- Organize and maintain supplies in a clean, orderly fashion.
- Follow a systematic procedure.
- Perform the facial massage properly.

Actions to Avoid

- harming or scratching the skin
- excessive or rough massage
- product in the client's eyes

- using towels that are too hot

- breathing into the client's face

- not being careful or sanitary

- disinterest in the client's skin problems or conversation

- leaving excess product on the skin

- excessive talking that does not facilitate client relaxation

- leaving the chair to obtain materials or supplies

- heavy, rough, or cold hands

Vibratory Facial

When using an electric massager on the face, avoid heavy contact with the client's skin. Delicate areas around the nose and upper cheek require a special technique using both of the barber's hands. The right-handed barber will attach the massager to his or her right hand. The left hand is placed on the client's skin. Next, the barber places his or her right hand on top of the left and the vibrations travel through this hand to the client's skin. Direct contact with the barber's right hand can be made to less delicate areas such as the forehead and jaw line, but pressure still needs to be avoided.

! CAUTION

The vibrator should never be used when there is a known weakness of the heart or in cases of fever, abscesses, or skin inflammations.

 procedure no. 7

Using an Electric Massager

The following steps outline massage movements to use with an electric massager:

1. Adjust the massager on the right hand and place the fingertips of the left hand on the client's left nostril.

Place the vibrating right-hand fingers over the left-hand fingers to vibrate through the left hand.

2   Vibrate the skin with a few light up-and-down movements on the left side of the nose.

3   Gently slide the fingers along the upper cheek area and direct them toward the center of the forehead.

4   Place the vibrating right hand onto the skin and perform rotary movements toward the left temple. Pause for a moment.

5   Continue the rotary movements down along the jaw line toward the tip of the chin.

6   Vibrate from the chin back toward the cheek, using wider, firmer movements.

7   Continue with a slow, light stroke at the temple, around the left ear, over the jawbone, toward the center of the neck, and then below the chin.

8   Vibrate rotary movements over the neck, behind the ear, up to the temple, and then toward the center of the forehead.

9   Repeat steps 2 through 8 on the right side of the face.

10 Repeat steps 2 through 8 on both sides of the face again and proceed with step 5 of the vibratory facial procedure that follows.

▷ procedure no. 8

Vibratory Facial

The procedure for a vibratory facial is similar to the basic facial with minor variations. Again, we emphasize that the following procedure may be changed to conform with your shop's routine.

1 Prepare the client as for a basic facial.

2 Apply steam towels.

3 Apply massage cream.

4 Administer the massage using the electric massager as described in the preceding section.

5 Apply cleansing cream with light hand manipulations.

6 Remove cleansing cream with a warm towel.

7 Follow with a mild witch hazel steam.

8 Apply one or two cool towels.

9 Apply a moisturizing face lotion.

10 Dry thoroughly and apply powder if desired.

Rules for Using an Electric Massager

- Regulate the number of vibrations to avoid overstimulation.

- Do not use the vibrator for too long in any one spot.

- Vary the amount of pressure in accordance with the results desired.

- Do not use a vibrator over the upper lip, as the vibrations may cause discomfort.

- For soothing and relaxing effects, give very slow, light vibrations for a very short time.

- For stimulating effects, give light vibrations of moderate speed and time.

- To reduce fatty tissues, give moderate, fast vibrations with firm pressure.

Rolling Cream Facial

The facial massage most often identified with the barbershop is the rolling cream facial. The rolling cream facial is designed to cleanse and stimulate the skin. Due to the drying qualities of the rolling cream and the application process, this type of facial should be recommended only to clients with normal, oily, or thick skin. It should not be performed on skin that is dry, acne-prone, sensitive, or thin in texture.

▷ procedure no. 9

Rolling Cream Facial

1. Prepare the client.

2. Moderately steam the face with two or three warm towels.

3. Apply dabs of rolling cream to the chin, cheeks, and forehead. Dampen the fingertips of both hands with water and spread the cream evenly over the face and neck with a smooth, stroking movement.

4. Massage the face and neck with uniform, rotary, stroking and rubbing movements with the cushion tips of the fingers, until most of the cream has rolled off.

5. Apply a small amount of cleansing cream to the face and neck, using lighter manipulations.

6. Remove the cream with a warm towel.

7. Apply a witch hazel steam to the face and neck with one or more hot towels, following with one or two cool towels to close the pores.

8. Apply astringent or toner. Dry and powder the face and neck.

9. Finish as for a basic facial.

Facial for Dry Skin

Dry skin is caused by an insufficient flow of sebum from the sebaceous glands. The objective of a facial for dry skin is to help moisturize it. Dry-skin facials can be performed using infrared rays, galvanic current, or high-frequency current.

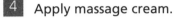 **procedure no. 10**

Dry-Skin Facial with Infrared Rays

1. Prepare the client as for a basic facial.

2. Apply cleansing cream; remove cream with a warm, moist towel.

3. Sponge the face with a mild tonic lotion.

4. Apply massage cream.

5. Apply lubricating oil, or eye cream, over and under the eyes.

6. Apply lubricating oil over the neck.

7. Cover the client's eyes with cotton pads moistened with witch hazel or a nonalcoholic freshener.

8. Expose the face and neck to infrared rays for not more than five minutes.

9. Perform massage manipulations three to five times.

10. Remove the massage cream and oil with tissues, or with a warm, moist towel.

11. Apply tonic lotion suitable for dry skin. Blot the face dry with tissues or a towel.

12. Apply moisturizer.

13. Complete and clean up as for a basic facial.

▷ procedure no. 11

Dry-Skin Facial with Galvanic Current

The procedure for giving a dry-skin facial with galvanic current is similar to the procedure for giving a dry-skin facial with infrared rays, with a few changes:

1. Repeat steps 1 through 4 of the procedure used with infrared rays.

2. Apply a thick layer of ionized, oil-free gel to the face and neck.

3. Apply negative galvanic current for five to seven minutes, to open the pores.

4. Reapply gel to the face and neck.

5. Apply positive galvanic current for four to six minutes, to close the pores.

6. Repeat steps 4 through 6 of the procedure used with infrared rays.

7. Repeat steps 9 through 13 of the procedure used with infrared rays.

▷ procedure no. 12

Dry-Skin Facial with Indirect High-Frequency Current

1. Follow steps 1 through 6 of the procedure for a facial with infrared rays.

2. Have client hold electrode in his right hand.

3. Perform manipulations, using the indirect method of applying high-frequency current, for 7 to 10 minutes.

Do not use tapping movements and do not lift hands from the client's skin.

4 Apply two or three cool towels to the face and neck.

5 Follow steps 10 to 13 of the procedure for a facial with infrared rays.

Facial for Oily Skin and Blackheads

Oily skin and/or blackheads are caused by hardened masses of sebum formed inside a follicle. The sebaceous material in the follicle darkens when exposed to oxygen, thus forming a blackhead.

 ## procedure no. 13

Oily Skin Facial

1 Prepare the client as for a basic facial.

2 Apply cleansing lotion and remove it with a warm, moist towel or facial sponges.

3 Place moistened eye pads on the client's eyes, then analyze the skin under a magnifying lamp.

4 Steam the face with three or four moist, warm towels, or a facial steamer, to open the pores.

5 Wear gloves and cover your fingertips with cotton and gently press out blackheads. Do not press so hard as to bruise the skin tissue.

6 Sponge the face with astringent or toner.

7   *Optional:* Cover the client's eyes with pads moistened with a mild astringent. Apply ultraviolet light over the skin for three to five minutes.

8   Apply massage cream suitable for the skin condition and perform massage manipulations.

9   Remove cream with a warm, moist towel, cotton pads, or facial sponges.

10 Moisten a cotton pledget with an astringent lotion. Apply it to the face and neck with upward and outward movements to constrict the pores. Blot the excess moisture with tissues. For male clients with beards, use downward and outward movements in the same direction as the hair growth.

11 Apply moisturizer or protective lotion according to skin type.

12 Complete and clean up as for basic facial procedure.

> ■ TECH TERM
>
> A *pledget* is a small square of cotton used for applying products to the skin.

Facial for Acne

Acne is a disorder of the sebaceous glands and serious cases require medical direction. If the client is under medical care, the role of the barber is to perform facial treatments as prescribed by the client's physician. If in doubt, contact the physician directly. With a prescribed treatment plan, treatment of acne conditions by barbers should be limited to the following procedures:

- reduction of oily skin by local and topical applications
- removal of blackheads using proper procedures
- cleansing of the skin
- application of medicated and/or prescribed preparations

▷ procedure no. 14

Acne Facial

Because acne contains infectious matter, it is advisable to use rubber or latex gloves and disposable materials such as cotton cleansing pads.

1 Prepare the client as for a basic facial.

2 Cleanse the client's face as in a basic facial.

3 Place cotton eye pads over the client's eyes; then analyze the skin under the magnifying lamp.

4 Apply warm, moist towels to the face to open the pores for deep cleansing.

5 Extract comedones as in a facial for oily skin.

6 Cleanse the face with a cotton pad or sponge that has been sprinkled with astringent.

7 *Optional:* Apply high-frequency current with direct application over the affected area for up to five minutes. Or, cover the client's eyes with goggles and apply ultraviolet light over the skin for three to five minutes for its germicidal effects.

8 Apply prescribed acne treatment cream if available. *Optional:* Leave the eye pads in place and apply infrared lamp for five to seven minutes to promote penetration of the treatment cream.

9 Leave the eye pads in place and apply a treatment mask that is suitable for the skin condition for 8 to 10 minutes.

10 Remove the mask with moist towels or sponges.

11 Apply astringent to the face with a wet cotton pad or sponge.

CAUTION

If high-frequency current is used as in step 7, use a nonalcoholic toner in place of the astringent.

CAUTION

Overexposure to ultraviolet rays can destroy skin tissue. Start with a two- or three-minute exposure time and gradually increase to seven or eight minutes.

 Apply protective fluid or special acne lotion.

13 Complete cleanup and sanitation procedures as for basic facial procedures.

Hot-Oil Mask

The hot-oil mask can be used for extremely dry, parched, and scaly skin that is prevalent during dry, hot, or windy weather. Although many commercially prepared products are on the market, some older clients may request this service to soften, smooth, and stimulate skin tissues.

Formula for a Hot-Oil Mask

2 tablespoons of olive oil

1 tablespoon of castor oil (refined grade)

1/4 teaspoon of glycerin

Mix the oils in a small container and warm.

 procedure no. 15

Hot-Oil Mask

1 Prepare the client as for a basic facial.

2 Prepare the mask. Saturate cotton pads (4″ × 4″) or an 18-inch square of gauze with the warm oil mixture.

3 Follow steps 1 through 11 as in a basic facial.

4 After the manipulations, do not remove the massage cream. Place eye pads and gauze in position over the face.

5 Use red dermal light or an infrared lamp for 8 to 10 minutes.

6 Remove the mask and cream.

7 Finish as for a basic facial.

THE NEXT STEP

Today's professional barber is being called upon to perform more than just the traditional hair cut. As a result of the image-concious, fast-paced world we live in, more and more men are looking for a barber who offers a full line of skin and hair care services. In the preceding section, facial massage and treatments were discussed. When offered in a clean, safe, and comfortable manner, these services will improve a client's appearance, relax him, and rejuvenate his skin. Other services that will promote a client's relaxation and improve his appearance include a professional shave and facial hair design. In the next section, a step-by-step guide of how to perform each is provided.

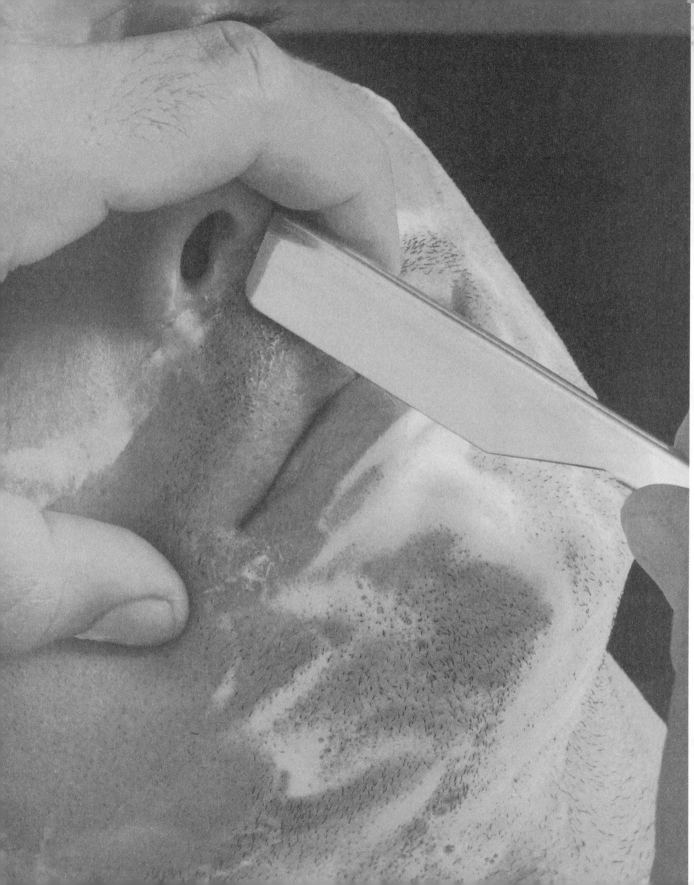

SHAVING AND FACIAL HAIR DESIGN

2

Although the advance of safety and electric razors over the past century has made it more convenient for men to shave at home, there will always be those clients who choose to indulge in a barbershop shave on an occasional, if not regular, basis. A full facial shave, complete with hot towels, lotions, and massage, is one of the most relaxing yet rejuvenating services that men can enjoy in the barbershop.

Shaving is an art. As such, it requires careful attention, skill, and practice to perfect. It is the professional barber's responsibility to learn the mechanics and perfect the art.

Note: It is critical that you read and study the entire shaving section before engaging in the performance of a facial shave.

■ TECH TERM

A *changeable blade straight razor* is a type of straight razor that uses changeable, disposable blades. A *conventional straight razor* is a razor made of a hardened steel blade that requires honing and stropping to produce a cutting edge.

■ | FUNDAMENTALS OF SHAVING

Shaving is one of the basic services performed in the barbershop. The objective of shaving is to remove the visible part of facial and neck hair without causing irritation to the skin. Professional barbers use a straight razor (changeable blade or conventional) and warm lather when shaving a client.

Certain general principles of shaving apply to all men. Because each individual is different, exceptions to these principles also exist that will require consideration. For example, the application of hot towels is a standard procedure in preparing the beard for shaving. Nevertheless, some clients may not tolerate a hot towel on their skin. Other individual characteristics such as hair texture, hair growth patterns, and product sensitivity are variables that barbers must consider and make educated judgments about before proceeding with the shave service.

General Sanitation and Safety Precautions of Shaving

Some general rules to be observed when shaving include the following:

- Always sanitize tools before use.

- Once the client is in position for the shave, lock the chair.

- Always use a forward sawing motion with the point of the blade in the lead when using a conventional straight razor. Use a gentle scraping motion with changeable blade razors.

- Always observe the hair growth pattern and shave with it, not against it.

- Heavy beard growth requires more care in the lathering process and more steam towels than usual to effectively prepare it for the shave.

- Lather against the grain gently to place the facial hair in a position to be shaved.

- Lather should be neatly applied to the areas to be shaved and replaced as necessary.

- The fingers of the hand opposite the hand holding the razor should be kept dry in order to grasp, stretch, and hold the skin firmly during the shave service.

- Hot towels should not be used on skin that is chapped or blistered from heat or cold, or on skin that is thin and sensitive.

- When astringents are too harsh for sensitive skin, pH-balanced fresheners or toners should be used.

■ TECH TERM

A *hone* is a sharpening block manufactured from rock or synthetic materials used to create a cutting edge on conventional straight razors.

■ TECH TERM

A *strop* is an elongated piece of leather or other material used to finish the edge of conventional straight razors to a smooth, whetted cutting edge.

- Clients that have an infection in the area to be shaved should not be served because doing so could spread the infection to other parts of the face or to the barber.

- Curly facial hair requires special care because its growth characteristics may cause problems if the shave isn't performed correctly. Ingrown hairs are often the result of improper hair removal by a razor, tweezers, or trimmer. Curly hair has the tendency to grow in a "looped" direction—as it grows out of the skin, it can bend back into the skin surface. Excessively close shaving with clippers, trimmers, or razors, coupled with excessive pressure, can damage skin to the point that new hair growth is trapped under the injured tissue. This can result in infected bumps on and under the skin surface (folliculitis), scar tissue, or the initiation of a keloid condition.

- Take special precautions when shaving beneath the lower lip, the lower part of the neck, and around the Adam's apple. These facial areas are usually the most tender and sensitive and are easily irritated by very close shaving.

- When small cuts and nicks occur, pat dry with a sterile cotton pledget and apply styptic powder.

- Keep the skin moist while shaving.

■ TECH TERM

A *keloid* is a thick scar resulting from excessive tissue growth.

! CAUTION

Never use a styptic pencil or other astringent that will come into contact with another person's face.

 STATE BOARD REGULATIONS

Some states may require the use of protective gloves while shaving a client. Be guided by your state barber board regulations.

Four Standard Shaving Positions and Strokes

The correct angle of cutting the beard with a straight razor is called the *cutting stroke.* To achieve the best cutting stroke, the razor must glide over the surface at an angle *with the grain of the hair.* It should be drawn in a forward movement with the point of the razor in the lead.

The first step in performing a professional shave is to master the fundamentals of handling the razor. This includes learning how to open and close the razor without injury. To open the razor, grasp the back of the razor's blade between the thumb and index finger of the dominant hand while holding the handle with the opposite thumb and index finger. As the blade and handle separate by way of the pivot (Figure 39), reposition the little finger of the dominant hand to rest on the tang as the handle is placed in an upward position (Figure 40). When closing the razor, be careful that the cutting edge does not strike the handle (Figure 41).

To shave the face with ease and efficiency, the barber employs four standard positions and strokes:

- Freehand position and stroke
- Backhand position and stroke
- Reverse freehand position and stroke
- Reverse backhand position and stroke

Each of the four standard shaving positions and strokes requires consideration and practice of the following:

CAUTION

Always handle razors with extreme care. A warped or loose razor handle may cause the blade to pass through to the fingers.

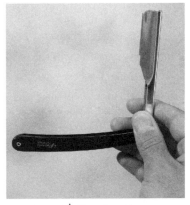

FIGURE 39 | Opening the razor.

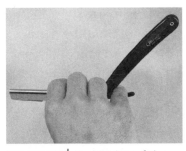

FIGURE 40 | Positioning of the little finger.

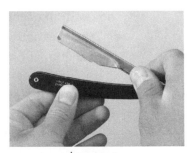

FIGURE 41 | Close the razor carefully.

reminder

Be careful that the cutting edge does not strike the handle when closing the razor.

STATE BOARD REGULATIONS

Some states prohibit the use of conventional straight razors and allow only changeable-blade razors. Be guided by your state barber board rules and regulations.

1. When to use a particular shaving stroke

2. How to hold the razor for each stroke
   a. The position of the right hand in relation to the razor
   b. The position of the left hand in relation to the razor

3. How to stroke the razor

Note: If using a conventional straight razor, review the proper honing and stropping methods before learning each shaving stroke.

Mastering the correct hand and finger placement, razor control, and cutting strokes requires practice. Practice the following procedures to become comfortable and proficient with a straight razor. The holding positions and strokes that barbers most often employ during the shave service are the freehand, backhand, reverse freehand, and reverse backhand.

▷ procedure no. 16

Freehand Position and Stroke

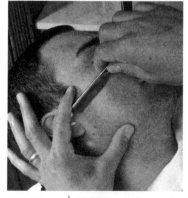

FIGURE 42 | Holding position of razor for freehand stroke.

1 How to hold the razor:

The position of the right hand is as follows:
a. Take the razor in the right hand. Hold the handle of the razor between the third and fourth fingers, with the tip of the small finger resting on the tip of the tang of the razor. The thumb should rest on the side of the shank near the shoulder of the blade. The third finger lies at the pivot of the shank and the handle, with the first and second fingers in front of it on the back of the shank (Figure 42).

b. Raise the right elbow to be level with the shoulder. This is the position used in the arm movement.

The position of the left hand is as follows:

c. Keep the fingers of the left hand dry in order to prevent them from slipping on the face.

d. Use the left hand to stretch the skin under the razor (Figure 43).

2 How to perform the freehand stroke in the freehand position:

a. Use a gliding stroke, toward you.

b. Direct the stroke toward the point of the razor in a forward, sawing movement.

3 When to use the freehand stroke:

The freehand position and stroke is used in 6 of the 14 shaving areas. See Nos. 1, 3, 4, 7, 11, and 12 in Figures 44 through 46. Please refer to your state's barbering regulations when identifying the numbered shaving areas of 6, 7, and 8 illustrated in Figure 44.

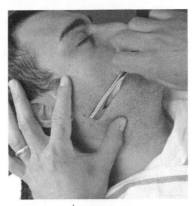

FIGURE 43 | Stretch the skin gently with the left hand.

 STATE BOARD REGULATIONS

Refer to your state barber board rules and regulations when identifying shaving areas 6, 7, and 8.

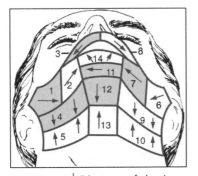

FIGURE 44 | Diagram of shaving areas of the face.

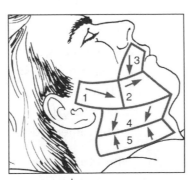

FIGURE 45 | Diagram of shaving areas on the right side of the face.

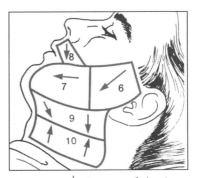

FIGURE 46 | Diagram of shaving areas on the left side of the face.

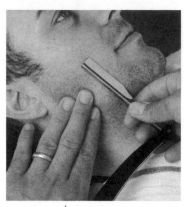

FIGURE 47 | Backhand holding position.

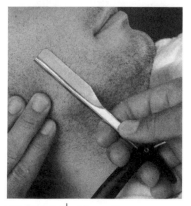

FIGURE 48 | Alternative backhand holding position.

 procedure no. 17

Backhand Position and Stroke

1 How to hold the razor:

The position of the right hand is as follows:
a. Hold the shank of the razor firmly with the handle bent slightly back.
b. Rest the shank of the razor on the first two joints of the first three fingers. Hold the thumb on the underside of the shank. Rest the end of the tang inside the first joint of the third finger, as in Figure 47. The little finger remains idle. An alternative holding position is shown in Figure 48.
c. Turn the back of the hand away from you and bend the wrist slightly downward. Then raise the elbow so that you can move the arm freely. This is the position used for the backhand stroke with the arm movement. Some practitioners prefer to use a wrist movement, in which case the arm is not held as high.

The position of the left hand is as follows:
d. Keep the fingers of the left hand dry in order to prevent them from slipping.
e. Stretch the skin under the razor.

2 How to perform the backhand stroke in the backhand position:
a. Use a gliding stroke away from you.
b. Direct the stroke toward the point of the razor in a forward, sawing movement or gentle scraping movement, depending on the type of razor used.

3 When to use the backhand stroke:

The backhand stroke is used in 4 of the 14 basic shaving areas. See Nos. 2, 6, 8, and 9 in Figures 44 through 46 and, if preferred, in area 12.

procedure no. 18

Reverse Freehand Position and Stroke

The reverse freehand stroke hand and razor position is similar to the freehand stroke. The stroke movement, however, is performed in an upward rather than a downward direction.

1 How to hold the razor:

The position of the right hand is as follows:
a. Hold the razor firmly, as in a freehand position.
b. Turn the hand slightly toward you so that the razor edge is turned upward (Figure 49).

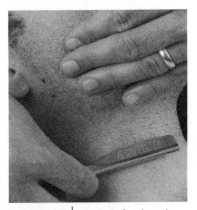

FIGURE 49 │ Reverse freehand stroke.

The position of the left hand is as follows:
c. Keep the hand dry and use it to pull the skin taut under the razor.
d. The left hand will be the hand closest to the barber's body in this position.

2 How to perform the reverse freehand stroke in the reverse freehand position:
a. Use an upward, semi-arc stroke toward you.
b. The movement is from the elbow to the hand, with a slight twist of the wrist.

3 When to use the reverse freehand stroke:

The reverse freehand stroke is used in 4 of the 14 basic shaving areas. See Nos. 5, 10, 13, and 14 in Figures 44 through 46.

procedure no. 19

Reverse Backhand Position and Stroke

The reverse backhand position and stroke require diligent practice to master. The holding position of the razor is the same as that for the backhand stroke except the elbow is positioned downward and the forearm is held upward. When using this stroke, make short cutting strokes in an upward (or downward, depending on shaving area) and slightly outward direction.

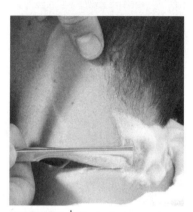

FIGURE 50 | Neck shave on the left side with reverse backhand stroke.

reminder

The beard should be shaved at an angle with the grain of the hair; therefore, the barber must determine when the reverse hand positions and strokes are the correct procedure for shaving the client's beard. For example: When the hair in shaving area No. 5 grows downward, the freehand stroke is a better choice than the reverse freehand stroke.

1 How to hold the razor:

The position of the right hand is as follows:
a. Hold the razor firmly, as in the backhand position.
b. Turn the palm of the hand to the right so that it faces upward.
c. Drop the elbow close to the side.

The position of the left hand is as follows:
d. Position the left hand so as to be able to draw the skin taut under the razor.
e. The barber's hand will be positioned above the razor (Figure 50).

2 How to perform the reverse backhand stroke in the reverse backhand position:
a. Use a short gliding stroke, directed downward toward the point of the razor.
b. Proceed with short cutting strokes directed downward and slightly outward.

3 When to use the reverse backhand stroke:
The reverse backhand stroke is used for making the left sideburn outline and for shaving the left side behind the ear during a neck shave while the client is sitting in an upright position.

The cutting strokes described in the preceding section illustrate the holding and stroking positions that should be employed by the right-handed barber. The left-handed barber will need to reverse the starting position as outlined in Table 7.

Table 7		SHAVING MOVEMENTS FOR LEFT-HANDED AND RIGHT-HANDED BARBERS		
MOVEMENT	**AREA OF FACE FOR A LEFT-HANDED BARBER**	**POSITION**	**DIRECTION**	**AREA OF FACE FOR A RIGHT-HANDED BARBER**
1	Left sideburn	Freehand	Down	Right sideburn
2	Left side of cheek	Backhand	Down	Right side of cheek
3	Left upper lip	Freehand	Down	Right upper lip
4	Left side below jaw	Freehand	Down	Right side below jaw
5	Left side of neck	Reverse freehand	Up	Right side of neck
6	Right upper lip	Backhand	Down	Left sideburn
7	Right sideburn	Freehand	Down	Left side of cheek
8	Right side of cheek	Backhand	Down	Left upper lip
9	Right side below jaw	Backhand	Down	Left side below jaw
10	Right side of neck	Reverse freehand	Up	Left side of neck
11	Across chin R. to L.	Freehand	Across	Across chin L. to R.
12	Below chin	Freehand or Backhand	Down	Below chin
13	Middle of neck	Reverse freehand	Up	Middle of neck
14	Lower lip	Reverse freehand	Up	Lower lip

The Professional Shave

A professional shave consists of preparation, shaving, and finishing. The following procedures explain these steps in detail.

▷ procedure no. 20

How to Prepare a Client for Shaving

1   Seat the client comfortably in the chair.

2   Ask the client to loosen his collar. Lay the drape over the client's clothing from the front.

3   Change the headrest cover and adjust it to the proper height.

4   Lower, adjust, and lock the chair to the proper height and level.

5   Wash your hands with soap and warm water, and dry them thoroughly.

6   Unfold a clean towel, and lay it diagonally across the client's chest.

7   Tuck one corner of the towel along the right side of the client's neck, securing the edge tucked inside the neckband with a sliding movement of the forefinger of the left hand. The lower end of the towel is crossed over to the other side of the client's neck and tucked under the neckband, with a similar sliding motion. A second towel or paper strip that is used during the shave to wipe the razor clean of shaving cream and facial hair should be tucked into the neckband and laid across the chest (Figure 51).

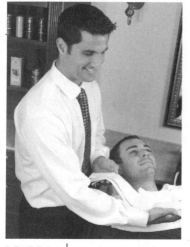

FIGURE 51 | Draping second towel across the chest.

▷ procedure no. 21

How to Prepare the Face for Shaving

Lathering and steaming the face are very important steps in preparing the skin for shaving. *Lathering* serves to cleanse the skin, soften the hair, hold the hair in an upright position, and create a smooth, flat surface over which the razor can glide more effectively. *Steaming* the face helps to soften the hair cuticle, provides lubrication by stimulating the action of the oil glands, and relaxes the client. If the client has a mustache, trim and shape it prior to the shave service to prepare it for finish work with the razor.

The face is prepared for shaving as follows:

1. Warm shaving lather is usually prepared in an electric latherizer. Transfer a quantity of lather into the hand and spread it evenly over the bearded areas of the face and neck to be shaved.

2. Use a rotary movement to briskly rub lather into the bearded area with the cushion tips of the fingers. Start at the neck and rub lather up to the right side of the face. Then gently turn the head with the left hand by lightly grasping the top of the head or the back of the head near the crown. Rub lather on the other side of the face and continue lathering until the bearded areas are covered. Rubbing time is from one to two minutes, depending on the stiffness and density of the beard (Figure 52).

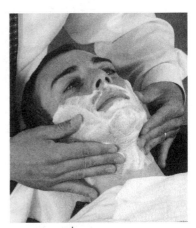

FIGURE 52 │ Use rotary movements to later the face.

3. To prepare a steam towel, fold a clean towel in half lengthwise (Figure 53). Then fold it in half again by bringing both ends of the towel together (Figure 54).

4. Place the folded towel under a stream of hot water or wrap it around the faucet or hose spray, until it becomes thoroughly saturated and heated (Figure 55).

   Note: *Thoroughly disinfect the sink, hose, and spray nozzle prior to preparing the steam towel.*

5. Wring out the towel.

6. Standing behind the client, position the steam towel in front of the chin area. Unfold the towel, holding it by the ends. Place the center of the towel over the client's mouth, under the chin, and across the lower part of the neck (Figure 56).

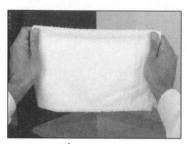

FIGURE 53 | Step 1: Fold a clean towel in half, lengthwise.

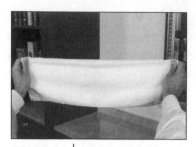

FIGURE 54 | Step 2: Fold the towel in half again.

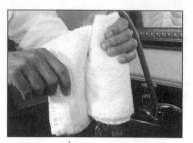

FIGURE 55 | Step 3: Wrap the towel around a stream of hot water.

! **CAUTION**

Do not use a hot steam towel if the skin is sensitive, irritated, chapped, or blistered.

Carefully wrap the towel around the face, leaving the nostrils exposed. Finally, fold the ends over each other on the forehead, covering the eyes (Figure 57). Repeat the steaming process if the beard is extremely coarse and/or dense.

7 While the steam towel is on the client's face, strop the razor (if using a conventional straight razor) and immerse it in sanitizing solution.

Note: New blades for changeable-blade razors do not guarantee a sanitized blade. Sanitize this style of razor as well. Then wipe the razor dry on a clean towel, and place it in a dry sanitizer or clean, closed container until ready for use.

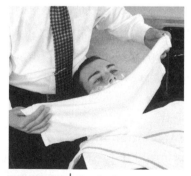

FIGURE 56 | Apply the steam towel.

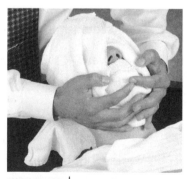

FIGURE 57 | Wrap the towel around the face, leaving the nostrils exposed.

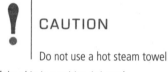

8 Remove the steam towel and wipe the lather off in one operation.

9 Relather the beard, then wipe the soap from your hands.

10 Standing on the client's right side, begin the shave process.

procedure no. 22

Position and Strokes in Shaving

Razor strokes should be correct and systematic. Proper coordination of both hands is necessary. While the right hand holds and strokes the razor, the fingers of the left hand gently stretch the skin area that is being shaved. Taut skin allows the beard hair to be cut more easily. Loose skin tends to push out in front of the razor and can result in cuts or nicks. Stretching the skin too tightly, however, will cause irritation. The skin must be held firmly, neither too loosely nor too tightly, to create a correct shaving surface for the razor. To prevent slipping, use alum block to help keep the fingers of the left hand dry at all times.

TECH TERM

Alum block consists of a double sulfate of ammonium or a univalent metal (sodium or potassium) and a trivalent metal (aluminum, iron, or chromium) and is used as an astringent; in powder form, it is used to stop the bleeding of minor skin wounds such as shaving nicks.

Shaving Area No. 1

Freehand stroke. Standing at the right side of the chair, gently turn the client's face to the left. With the second finger of the left hand, remove the lather from the hairline. Hold the razor as for a freehand stroke and gently stretch the skin from behind the razor. Beginning at the hairline on the right side, shave downward toward the jawbone with a gliding, cutting stroke from point to heel of the razor (Figure 58).

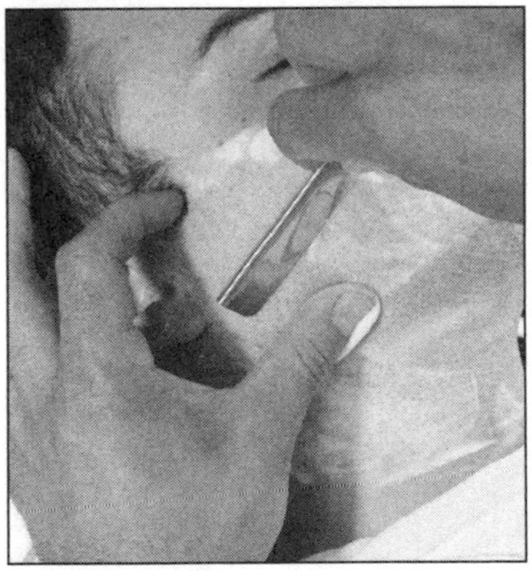

FIGURE 58 | Shaving area No. 1: freehand stroke.

Shaving Area No. 2

Backhand stroke. Remaining in the same position, wipe the razor clean on lather paper. Hold the razor as for a backhand stroke;

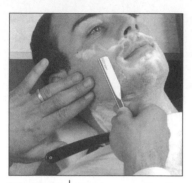

FIGURE 59 | Shaving area No. 2: backhand stroke.

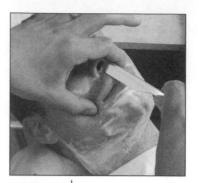

FIGURE 60 | Shaving area No. 3: freehand stroke.

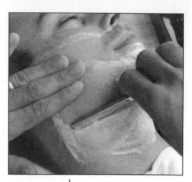

FIGURE 61 | Shaving area No. 4: freehand stroke.

use a diagonal stroke from point to heel and shave the right side of the face (Figure 59).

Shaving Area No. 3

Freehand stroke. Maintaining the same position, wipe the razor clean. Holding it in the same manner as for a freehand stroke, shave underneath the nostrils and over the right side of the upper lip, using the fingers of the left hand to stretch the underlying skin. When shaving underneath the nostril, slightly lift the tip of the nose, taking care not to interfere with breathing. To stretch the upper lip, place the fingers of the left hand against the nose, while holding the thumb below the lower corner of the lip (Figure 60). If the client has a mustache, shave the outline with the razor at this time.

Shaving Area No. 4

Freehand stroke. Start at the level of the chin and shave that portion below the jawbone down to the change in the grain of the beard. Be sure to hold the skin taut between the thumb and fingers of the left hand (Figure 61).

Shaving Area No. 5

Reverse freehand stroke. Move behind the chair. Hold the razor as for a reverse freehand stroke. Shave the remainder of the beard

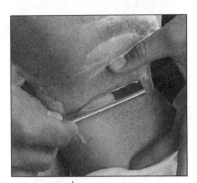

FIGURE 62 | Shaving area No. 5: reverse freehand stroke.

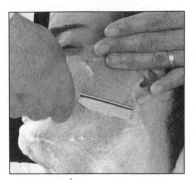

FIGURE 63 | Shaving area No. 6: backhand stroke.

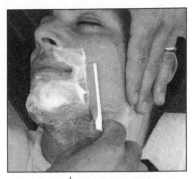

FIGURE 64 | Shaving area No. 7: freehand stroke.

upward with the grain (Figure 62). This movement completes shaving of the right side of the face.

Shaving Area No. 6

Backhand stroke. Stand slightly back from the client. Gently turn the face to the right. Relather the left side of the face. Using the thumb, wipe lather from the hairline. Stretch the skin with the fingers of the left hand and shave downward to the lower part of the ear, and slightly forward on the face (Figure 63).

Note: The skin must be stretched taut to prevent the razor from digging in along the ear.

Shaving Area No. 7

Freehand stroke. Wipe off the razor. Stand to the client's right. Hold the razor as for a freehand stroke. Shave downward on the left side of the face toward the jawbone and point of the chin (Figure 64).

Shaving Area No. 8

Backhand stroke. Wipe the razor clean and strop if necessary. Stand to the right side of the client and turn the client's face upward, so that you can shave the left upper lip. Hold the razor as

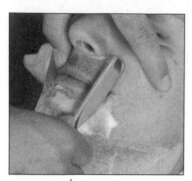

FIGURE 65 | Shaving area No. 8: backhand stroke.

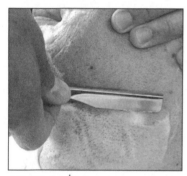

FIGURE 66 | Shaving area No. 9: backhand stroke.

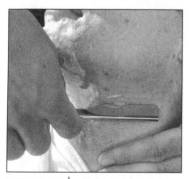

FIGURE 67 | Shaving area No. 10: reverse freehand stroke.

for a backhand stroke. While gently pushing the tip of the nose to the right with the thumb and fingers of the left hand, shave the left side of upper lip (Figure 65).

Shaving Area No. 9

Backhand stroke. Wipe off the razor. Maintaining the same position, hold the razor as for the backhand stroke. With the fingers of the left hand stretching the skin, shave downward to a point where the grain of the beard changes on the neck (Figure 66).

Shaving Area No. 10

Reverse freehand stroke. Wipe off the razor. Stand slightly back from the client. Hold the razor as for the reverse freehand stroke. Stretching the skin with the left hand, shave the left side of the neck upward (Figure 67).

Shaving Area No. 11

Freehand stroke. Stand at the client's side and turn the head so the face is pointing up. Holding the razor as for the freehand stroke, shave across the upper part of the chin. Continue shaving across the chin until it has been shaved to a point below the jawbone. The skin is stretched with the left hand (Figure 68).

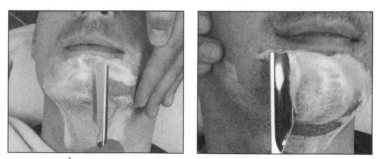

FIGURE 68 | Shaving area No. 11: freehand stroke.

Shaving Area No. 12

Freehand stroke. Stretch the skin with the left hand and shave the area just below the chin until the change in the grain of the beard is reached (Figure 69). *Alternate method:* Some barbers prefer to use the backhand stroke in shaving area No. 12.

Shaving Area No. 13

Reverse freehand stroke. Move behind the chair. Hold the razor as for the reverse freehand stroke. Stretch the skin below the chin toward the sides of the neck and shave upward along the sides of the Adam's apple on a slight diagonal to prevent nicks on the lower part of the neck (Figure 70).

Shaving Area No. 14

Reverse freehand stroke. Remain behind the chair. Shave upward from the chin toward the lower lip with a few, short reverse freehand strokes (Figure 71). Wipe off the razor and discard the towel or paper strip.

The Once-Over Shave

The once-over shave requires less time for a complete and even shave. To perform a once-over shave, shave a few more

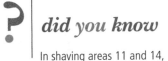

did you know

In shaving areas 11 and 14, the client can help to stretch the skin if he rolls his bottom lip slightly over his bottom teeth. This is known as *balling-the-chin.*

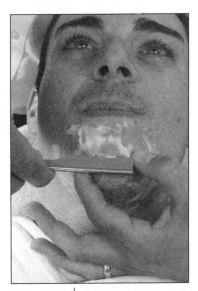

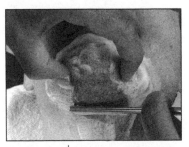

FIGURE 69 | Shaving area No. 12: freehand stroke.

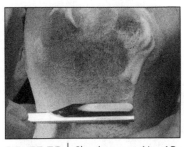

FIGURE 70 | Shaving area No. 13: reverse freehand stroke.

FIGURE 71 | Shaving area No. 14: reverse freehand stroke.

strokes *across the grain* while completing each shaving movement. This will assure a complete and even shave with a single lathering.

The Close Shave

Close shaving is the practice of shaving the beard *against the grain* of the hair during the second-time-over phase of the shave. This practice is undesirable because it may irritate the skin and lead to infection or ingrown hairs. For this reason, barbers and barber-stylists do not traditionally employ close shaving methods. However, should the client request it, first remove all traces of lather with a steam towel. Turn the towel over and place it on the face. After removing the steam towel, remoisten the bearded part of the face and proceed with the second-time-over shave. Use the freehand and reverse freehand strokes in this process.

Stand slightly behind the client. With a freehand stroke, shave the right side of the face. Stroking the grain of the beard sideways, shave the upper lip and work downward to the lower jawbone. Shave the lower part of the neck with a reverse freehand stroke and follow the grain of the beard.

Next, turn the client's face toward you. With a freehand stroke, shave the left side of the face. Stroking the grain of the beard sideways, shave from the ear toward the tip of the nose. When finished, wipe off the razor on lather paper, a neck strip, or a paper towel. Discard all soiled papers in a closed container.

▷ procedure no. 23

Final Steps of the Facial Shave

The final steps in shaving require attention to a number of important details.

1. Following the shave, apply light facial cream or moisturizing lotion with effleurage massage movements.

2. Prepare a moderately warm towel and apply it over the face.

   Note: A complete facial treatment may be performed at this time if the client desires the service.

3. Remove the towel from the face.

4. Apply a toner or other mild astringent using cotton pledgets or soft tissue. Pat gently; do not wipe or scrape against the skin.

5. Remove the towel from the client's chest and position yourself behind the chair.

6. Spread the towel over the client's face. Pat dry the lower part of the face, then the upper part. Remove the towel and fan the face dry.

7. Move to the right side of the chair and wrap a clean dry towel around your hand, as described in Procedure No. 24.

8. Sprinkle a small amount of talcum powder on the towel and apply evenly to the face.

9. Slowly raise the chair to an upright position.

10. Perform a neck shave if requested, as described in Procedure No. 25.

11. Comb the hair neatly as desired.

12. Wipe off loose hair, lather, or powder from the client's face and clothing. Proceed with mustache trim if not performed before shave service. Remove draping.

> **! CAUTION**
>
> Avoid excessively hot steam towels, as the skin may be sensitive after the shave service.

▶ procedure no. 24

Towel Wrap

Properly trained barbers and barber-stylists know how to wrap a towel around the hand with ease and skill for the purposes of:

- ◻ cleansing and drying the face.

- ◻ applying powder to the face.

- ◻ removing all traces of powder, lather, and loose hair from the face, neck, and forehead.

Practice the towel-wrapping methods illustrated in Figures 72 to 82 before beginning a facial shave service. Figures 72 to 74 show one method of wrapping a cotton towel around the hand; Figures 75 to 82 illustrate wrapping with a paper barber's towel. Either wrapping method can also be used with a flat-weave cotton towel.

Cloth towel wrap: Grasp towel lengthwise (Figure 72). Holding your right hand in front of you, draw the upper edge of the towel across the palm of the right hand; then grasp the towel ends and twist (Figure 73). Wrap the twisted ends of the towel around the back of the hand and bring them over the inside of the wrist (Figure 74). Hold the ends of the towel while in use to prevent them from flapping in the client's face.

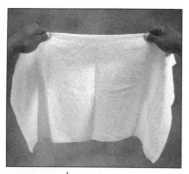

FIGURE 72 | Grasp towel lengthwise.

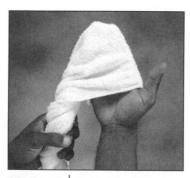

FIGURE 73 | Draw towel over palm and twist the ends.

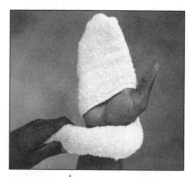

FIGURE 74 | Wrap twisted towel ends around back of hand and across the wrist.

Paper towel wrap: Grasp the towel lengthwise (Figure 75). Fold down the top third of the towel toward you (Figure 76). Holding the towel at one end, insert the two middle fingers into the fold (Figure 77); maintain your grip on the towel with the thumb, index finger, and fourth finger. Bring the top edge around the back of the hand and secure with the fourth finger (Figures 78a and 78b). Grasp the towel end and shift to a diagonal position (Figure 79). Wrap the remaining towel length around the back of the hand and insert the thumb into the fold (Figure 80). Continue the wrapping motion around the thumb (Figure 81). Tuck the towel end into the wrap at the back of the hand (Figure 82).

▷ procedure no. 25

The Neck Shave

The neck shave follows a haircut and involves shaving the neckline on both sides of the neck below the ears and across the nape, if desired and necessary.

Raise the chair slowly to an upright position and tuck the towel around the back of the neck. Leave the drape and towel loose enough to facilitate access to the sides and bottom of the neckline. Tuck a neck strip or paper toweling into the neckline of the drape for wiping the blade of lather. Apply lather. Shave the neckline, first at the right side using a freehand stroke, and then at the left side using a reverse backhand stroke, as described in Procedure No. 19 (Figures 83 and 84). Use a freehand stroke to shave the nape area as desired (Figure 85).

Clean the shaven part of the neckline with toweling or a neck strip moistened with witch hazel, antiseptic, or warm water. Remove the towel from around the neck and dry thoroughly. (This is the time to suggest a leave-in scalp treatment or hair tonic.) Position yourself behind the chair, replace the towel around the client's neck, and comb or style the hair as desired by the client.

i **FYI**

Sometimes a client requests a neck shave following a facial shave in order to maintain a well-groomed appearance between haircuts.

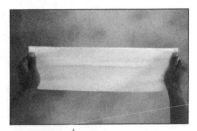

FIGURE 75 | Grasp the towel lengthwise.

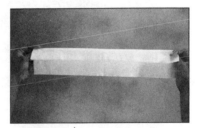

FIGURE 76 | Fold down top third of towel.

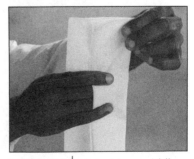

FIGURE 77 | Insert two middle fingers into the fold.

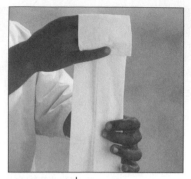

FIGURE 78A | Bring top edge around hand and secure with fourth finger.

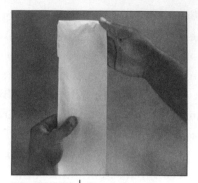

FIGURE 78B | Front view.

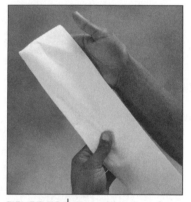

FIGURE 79 | Reposition towel diagonally.

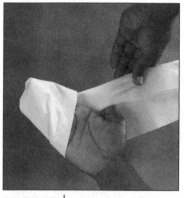

FIGURE 80 | Wrap hand and insert thumb into fold.

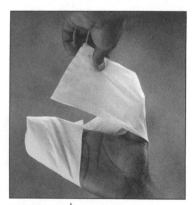

FIGURE 81 | Wrap the thumb.

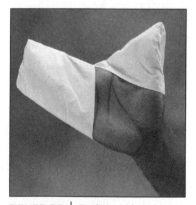

FIGURE 82 | Tuck towel end into wrap at back of hand.

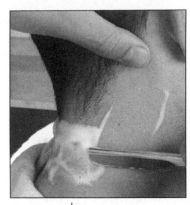

FIGURE 83 | Neck shave on the right side with freehand stroke.

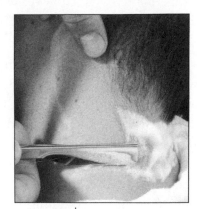

FIGURE 84 | Neck shave on the left side with reverse backhand stroke.

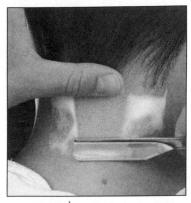

FIGURE 85 | Neck shave in the nape area with freehand stroke.

Take the towel from the back of the neck and fold it around the right hand. Remove all traces of powder and any loose hair. Discard the towel and remove the chair cloth from the client. Make out the price check and thank the client as it is handed to him.

Customer Satisfaction

Though there are many reasons why a client may find fault with the shave procedure, the most common are as follows:

- dull or rough razors
- unclean hands, towels, or shaving cloth
- cold fingers
- heavy touch
- poorly heated towels
- lather that is either too cold or too hot
- glaring overhead lights
- unshaven hair patches
- scraping the skin and close shaving
- offensive body odor or foul breath of the barber

INTRODUCTION TO FACIAL HAIR DESIGN

In addition to cutting and styling hair, barbers and barber-stylists should be able to offer clients a full range of services for grooming facial hair. Unlike in the past, men do not have to wait for fashion trends to decide to grow their mustaches or beards. Because today's style is one of individuality, barbers and barber-stylists should become proficient, or even specialists, in the design and trimming of men's facial hair. The client that wears a mustache and/or beard will frequent a shop that can provide both haircutting and facial hair services.

THE MUSTACHE

The mustache is worn primarily for personal adornment rather than utility and the wearer is usually very particular about how it is designed and maintained. Care, artistry, and sensitivity to the client's preferences are required for this service. Corrective shaping or redesign of the mustache by the barber helps clients with their daily maintenance and trimming at home until the next visit to the barbershop.

In addition to knowing how to trim and shape mustaches, barbers and barber-stylists should be able to understand and apply certain principles of mustache design.

Mustache Design

Choosing a suitable mustache design depends on the client's facial features, hair growth, and personal taste. As with hairstyling services, facial features are of primary importance in the selection process. The size of the mustache should correspond to the size of the features—such as a large design for heavy features, and a smaller design for fine, small facial features.

Important facial characteristics that help to determine the choice of mustache design include: the width of the mouth; size of the nose; shape of upper lip area; width of the cheeks, jaw, and chin; and the density of hair growth. As a general rule, be guided by the client's pattern of hair growth and avoid cutting into natural hairlines too deeply to minimize daily maintenance. Additional guidelines for mustache design and proportion are as follows:

- Large, coarse facial features: heavier looking mustache

- Prominent nose: medium to large mustache

- Long, narrow face: narrow to medium mustache

- Extra-large mouth: pyramid-shaped mustache

- Extra-small mouth: medium, short mustache

- Smallish, regular features: smaller, triangular mustache

- Wide mouth with prominent upper lip: heavier handlebar or large, divided mustache

- Round face with regular features: semi-square mustache

- Square face with prominent features: heavier, linear mustache with ends slightly curving downward

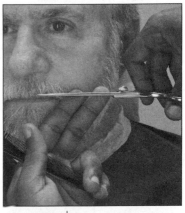

FIGURE 86 | Trimming mustache length with shears.

 ## procedure no. 26

Trimming a Mustache

1. Drape the client as for a haircut service.

2. Consult with the client regarding shape preferences.

3. Trim the mustache to the desired length with shears or outliner (Figures 86 and 87). Check for evenness of length at the corners of the mouth.

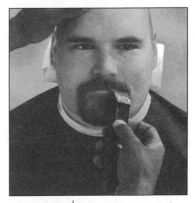

FIGURE 87 | Trimming mustache length with outliner.

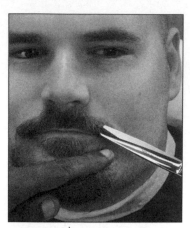

FIGURE 88 | Removing bulk using shears.

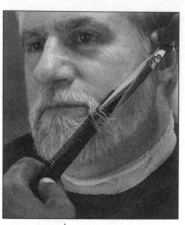

FIGURE 89 | Removing bulk using shear-over-comb method.

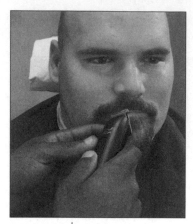

FIGURE 90 | Shaping the mustache with outliner.

 4 Remove bulk from the mustache using shears or shear-over-comb technique (Figures 88 and 89).

 5 Shape the mustache with a razor or outliner (Figure 90).

Additional mustache services that may be offered with a mustache trim include waxing mustache ends, penciling with temporary color, or coloring for overall color evenness or compatibility with scalp hair color.

THE BEARD

The purpose of a beard or goatee is to balance the facial features and correlate the proportions of face, head, and body. As with their mustaches, men are usually very particular about the design of their beards. Again, a careful approach, artistry, and sensitivity to the client's preferences are required for this service.

If the client is to receive a haircut service in addition to the beard trim, the decision must be made as to which service will be performed first. This is completely a matter of choice for the barber, as he or she will have his or her own reasons for doing so. Some barbers prefer to cut and style the hair prior to the beard trim so as to better balance the length and fullness of the beard with the hairstyle.

Beard Design

The correct shaping or redesign of the beard can emphasize pleasant facial features, minimize less desirable ones, and camouflage flaws. As with other hair design, it is important to develop a "good eye" for balance and proportion of the beard. Very few individuals have perfectly symmetrical face shapes, so barbers are usually challenged to create an illusion of symmetry. It may help the beginning barber to use an eyebrow pencil to draw the design and make any corrections prior to cutting the beard.

During the first trimming, it is advisable to leave the facial hair slightly longer than the desired end result. This helps to avoid cutting the hair too closely and leaves it long enough for retrimming toward the end of the beard-design service. Beard design and trimming is usually performed with a combination of the shears, comb, outliner (and/or clippers), and razor.

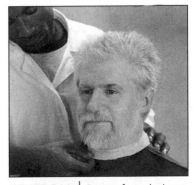

FIGURE 91A │ Drape for a haircut service.

▷ procedure no. 27

Trimming a Beard

1. Drape the client as for a haircut service (Figure 91a).

2. Consult with the client as to his desired design of the beard. Determine any preferences regarding length, density (thickness), and shape (Figure 91b).

3. With the client in an upright sitting position, use an eyebrow pencil to draw in the beard design

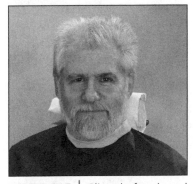

FIGURE 91B │ Client before beard trim.

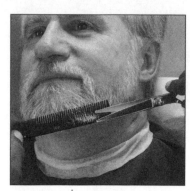

FIGURE 92 | Trim excess hair.

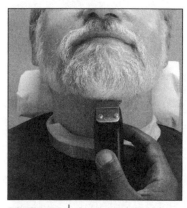

FIGURE 93 | Create a design line with outliner.

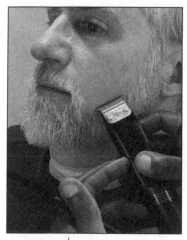

FIGURE 94 | Outline the cheek areas of the beard.

(optional). Confer with the client as to his preferences and approval.

 Adjust the headrest so the client's neck is supported while leaning his head back. The chair may also be reclined slightly or totally depending on your preference for reaching areas under the chin. Remember to check the proportion and shape of the beard when the client is returned to a sitting position.

 Place a towel underneath the chin to protect the client's neck from stray hairs (optional).

6 Trim excess hair with shears and comb (Figure 92).

7 Create a design line with the outliner. Start in the center directly under the chin and outline the under part of the beard (Figure 93). Work to the right side of the face up to the sideburn and ear area, then repeat for the left side.

8 Outline the cheek and upper areas of the beard, blending with the sideburn area (Figure 94).

9 Using the shear-over-comb technique, taper and blend the beard from the outlined areas up to just under the bottom lip, mustache, and cheek areas (Figure 95).

10 Trim and blend the mustache (Figure 96).

11 Apply steam towel, lather areas to be shaved, shave carefully at the outline, and wipe clean.

12 Return client to sitting position.

13 Wipe off any remaining lather or pencil marks. Apply after-shave lotion.

14 Check and retouch the beard with shears and outliner wherever necessary (Figure 97).

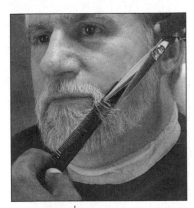

FIGURE 95 | Blend from outlined areas to mustache.

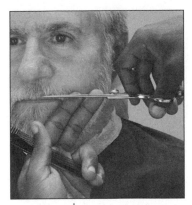

FIGURE 96 | Trim mustache.

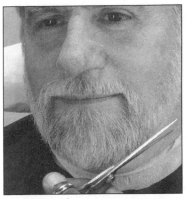

FIGURE 97 | Complete detail finish work on beard with shears.

 15 Style or cut the hair as needed for a finished look (Figure 98).

In some cases, your client may desire more than a beard trim . . . he may desire a whole new look! Such a request requires the barber to create a new beard design that complements and balances the structure of the client's face. Figures 99 to 106 show the progression of creating a new mustache and goatee design.

Clippers, Comb, and Outliner Method

Clippers may also be used for beard trimming, especially if one overall length is desired. Clipper-cut beard trims are most

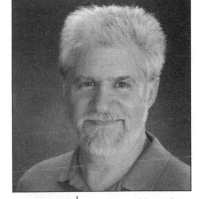

FIGURE 98 | Completed beard trim.

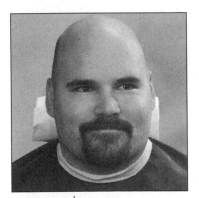

FIGURE 99 | Client before beard design

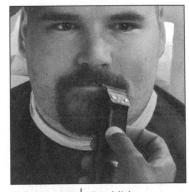

FIGURE 100 | Establish mustache length.

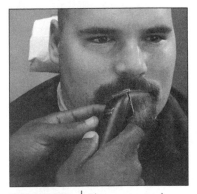

FIGURE 101 | Shape mustache from center to corner.

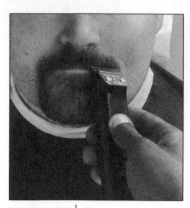

FIGURE 102 | Shape corner and ends of mustache.

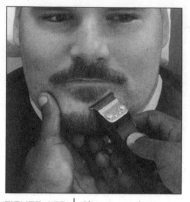

FIGURE 103 | Shape patch area under bottom lip (optional).

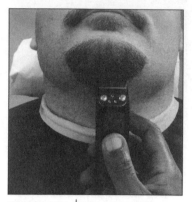

FIGURE 104 | Establish goatee design line.

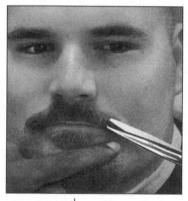

FIGURE 105 | Complete detail finish work on mustache, patch, and goatee with shears.

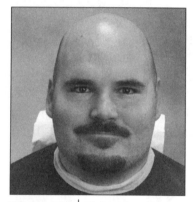

FIGURE 106 | Finished mustache and goatee design.

successful on clients whose beards are of an even density and texture. This is important to note because sometimes all-over even cutting may produce whorls or patches, especially in wavy hair.

Many beard lengths will require the use of a clipper comb attachment. Follow steps 1 through 8 of the previous procedure. Then proceed by choosing a comb attachment close to the length of the client's beard. If more than a light trim is required, select the next-shortest-length comb attachment. Repeat as required until desired length is achieved. Always follow up with shears for the final trimming.

FINAL THOUGHTS

In the preceding sections we have covered the fundamentals of facial massage, skin treatments, shaving, and facial hair design—important skills to master in order to meet the growing skin and hair care needs of your male clientele. We hope that after reading this book you find that offering these services proves physiologically and psychologically rewarding to your clients and professionally rewarding to you. We wish you the best of luck!

INDEX

Note: Page numbers followed by a "t" or an "f" indicate that the entry is included in a table or figure.

NOTES